TRANSFORMING THEMES

TRANSFORMING THEMES
Creative Perspectives on Therapeutic Interaction

Paul J. Leslie

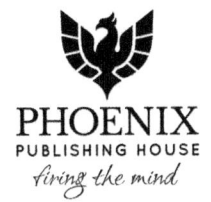

First published in 2021 by
Phoenix Publishing House Ltd
62 Bucknell Road
Bicester
Oxfordshire OX26 2DS

Copyright © 2021 by Paul J. Leslie

The right of Paul J. Leslie to be identified as the author of this work has been asserted in accordance with §§ 77 and 78 of the Copyright Design and Patents Act 1988.

All rights reserved. No part of this publication may be reproduced, stored in a retrieval system, or transmitted, in any form or by any means, electronic, mechanical, photocopying, recording, or otherwise, without the prior written permission of the publisher.

British Library Cataloguing in Publication Data

A C.I.P. for this book is available from the British Library

ISBN-13: 978-1-912691-98-2

Typeset by Medlar Publishing Solutions Pvt Ltd, India

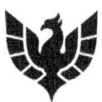

www.firingthemind.com

Contents

Acknowledgments — vii
About the author — ix
Introduction — xi

CHAPTER 1
Theme-oriented therapy — 1

CHAPTER 2
Psychotherapy as theme creation — 19

CHAPTER 3
Cocreating new themes — 49

CHAPTER 4
Thematic patterns and rituals — 71

CHAPTER 5
The soldier who was secretly a hippie — 91

CHAPTER 6
The heart of an artist 105

CHAPTER 7
The eccentric professor 119

References 131
Index 135

Acknowledgments

I would like to thank Kate Pearce and her wonderful team at Phoenix Publishing House who went out of their way to make the publishing process a delightful experience.

I also want to extend a big thank-you to my parents, Sue and Paul Leslie, who have consistently been my greatest supporters. I am forever grateful for their encouragement.

A very special thank-you to G.T. who continues to remind me that the best themes in life are those based on love, kindness, and compassion.

About the author

Paul J. Leslie is a psychotherapist, researcher, trainer, and author in Aiken, South Carolina. He specializes in resource-directed approaches to working with individuals and families. Paul is a licensed therapist and a National Board Certified Fellow in Hypnotherapy. He has a doctorate in counseling psychology and is presently the coordinator of the psychology program at Aiken Technical College. His website is www.drpaulleslie.com.

Introduction

A theme is a topic of discourse, a subject of discussion, or a dominating idea. Themes, as literary devices, give underlying meanings to an author's work. The theme of a story is its elemental message and the crucial beliefs that the author attempts to convey. Basically then, a theme is what a story means. Much of how we live our lives is rooted in the themes we use to explain our experiences, and like many works of literature, these themes are often hidden more deeply than we may think. They are the meanings that clients assign to their experiences, and the repetitive activation of these meanings creates overarching themes by which clients live their lives. Themes are self-reflexive and symbolic in nature, and serve to coordinate the internal processes of individuals, families, and even whole societies. Themes are what shape our relationships, values, and traditions, both individually and collectively. These dominating ideas are the higher-order metaphorical constructions that direct our lower-order thoughts, emotions, and behaviors, and if the theme is harmful, the clients' perceptions and reactions create what they perceive as their "problems."

This book is a pragmatic approach to helping clients to change, and the premise of this approach is that by assisting clients to change the limiting themes that they themselves have constructed, their own natural problem-solving abilities and healing resources can be activated. When therapists work from the higher-order of themes experiences, they have more freedom to increase their therapeutic opportunities. Since themes are a higher-order, therapists should not be restricted to only one specific theory or technique in their interventions. Any ethical action or directive on the part of the therapist may be used to shift the limiting themes in order to free clients and to help begin their self-healing. However, this requires collaborative experiential engagements between therapists and their clients that are spontaneous and experimental.

This method is not pathology-oriented, and the conversations will appear more improvisational, but these conversations provide openings which can lead clients out of their limited themes. From this perspective, client problems are not viewed as linear medical models with explanatory devices such as cognitive distortions, attachment disorders, or chemical imbalances. Instead clients have a "distressed" theme. This perspective shifts the focus of therapy from lower-order symptom pathology to the higher-order of constructed meanings. Since both therapist and client are then able to widen their possibilities of responding, they are not locked into rigid, standardized cause-and-effect interventions. As Papp and Imber-Black (1996) put it, "By identifying the overarching themes that operate repetitively at the individual, family, intergenerational, and socio-cultural levels, the therapist generates a new frame for viewing problems that spans many different levels of experience" (p. 6).

I began working with clients from a "theme" perspective many years ago when I noticed that my attempts to help clients move toward positive change using standardized, predetermined methods often came up short. To be fair, at times these methods could be effective, but I often found that they rarely led to real generative change in clients. Most psychotherapies work from a reductionist perspective in which complex issues are reduced down to their most simple components and from there specific techniques are applied to adjust that particular component. For example, suppose a client says that she has an "anger issue." From a reductionist perspective, the therapist will first attempt to find the root cause of the anger and then will try to change it using linear applications such as cognitive restructuring or exposure therapy. This can sometimes be effective, but it also ignores the higher-order of complexity that may be present.

As we will discover in this book, higher-order meanings often override lower-order thoughts, emotions, and actions. If change is only attempted at the lower orders of experience, then change may often be overpowered by the dominant meanings of the themes which guide clients' lives. It is only when higher-order complexity is taken into account that true generative change can begin to occur. This is sometimes a problem for therapists who have been trained to only respond to client issues from a reductionist theory. When higher-order complexity maintains the client's theme, and they do not respond to lower-order interventions, it is far too easy for therapists to label such clients as "resistant" or "unchangeable."

When we realize that therapy is a cooperative process that operates within certain agreed-upon themes, the process of therapy becomes less regimented and more spontaneous. Because the themes provided by clients are unique to each one of them, the quest for the perfect technique or theory that works every time will have to be abandoned. When changes are made to the problematic themes that clients bring with them to therapy, the very problems which initially appeared so entrenched will become much more malleable. Actions which took place in old themes can magically take on more empowering meanings in newer themes.

In contrast, working within problem-oriented themes will only continue to reinforce the original problem-oriented themes. As Ray and Keeney (1993) state,

> No matter what is said to the client, whether it be inquiring about the behavioral aspects of the problem, descriptions of attempted solutions, hypotheses about its origins, or professional categorizing and stigmatizing, if it contributes to the theme of the problem then the therapist is potentially helping the client stay stuck in a problem context. (p. 3)

Putting more emphasis on the themes which guide clients' emotions and behaviors requires that less emphasis will be placed on the minutiae that is commonly seen as important in therapy. Endless discussion on the topics of etiology and pathology are avoided since these are lower-order experiences that may not change higher-order perceptions.

My goal for this book is to introduce readers to a conceptual therapy that will give them more freedom and will enhance their interactions with their clients. Chapter 1 will first give an overview of how clients create the themes which lead them to seek psychotherapy. The importance of the awareness of the role of themes and contexts in therapy will be explored through perspectives taken from general semantics, cybernetic, epistemological, and postmodern philosophy.

Chapter 2 will explore how psychotherapy is a socially constructed cocreative process in which therapists and clients both agree upon the realities or themes which occur in the session. Research concerning successful "common factors" in therapy will show that technical and theoretical aspects in psychotherapy are not what primarily create change.

Chapter 3 will delve further into how the therapist and the client can cocreate outcomes and can shift focus to the higher-order resource-oriented themes over lower-order pathology-focused themes and thus create healing outcomes. Emphasis is placed on the need for therapists to direct sessions toward clients' strengths and resources while exhibiting greater levels of creativity, novelty, and improvisation when attempting to transform clients' limiting themes.

Chapter 4 provides an overview of applications for changing themes involving symbolic and unconscious methods that therapists can use when therapy has become stuck and hindered by the limits of language and attempts at conscious insight. Such tools as therapeutic tasks, rituals, metaphors, and pattern adjustments are covered.

Chapters 5, 6, and 7 are transcripts of therapy sessions with commentary. These demonstrate and explain how adjustments in the clients' themes can result in surprising levels of healing and positive outcomes. The names and other identifying information of clients in these transcripts and throughout the book have been changed to ensure confidentiality.

As I close this short introduction, I want to acknowledge the influences that have opened my eyes and altered my way of seeing therapeutic interaction. These influences came from my study of such sources as Korzybski (1958), Bateson (1972), Papp and Imber-Black (1996), O'Hanlon and Wilk (1987), Ray and Keeney (1993), and Gergen (2009). I honor their contributions and appreciate their desire to share their profound ideas.

CHAPTER 1

Theme-oriented therapy

Maggie and Anthony sat rigidly on the sofa in the counseling office, tightly holding each other's hands. The expression on their faces could best be described as devastated. As our session began, I quickly learned that these two people had suffered the worst event that any parent can ever experience. Their son had committed suicide in front of them and had died in their arms two weeks earlier. As we began our therapy session, their pain was palpable as they sobbed out feelings of regret and sorrow. They were reliving this tragedy daily. The theme of shock and horror reverberated around the office as these two people were seemingly locked into a never-ending theme of trauma and parental grief. Would they ever be able to move on with their lives after watching their son violently kill himself? Could they ever find peace within the all-encompassing theme of "The Parents Who Saw Too Much?"

Every day, therapists around the world will see their own version of Maggie and Anthony. Or they may see Jill and Bob who dwell in their own theme of anger and reprisal. Or they could see Sylvia who lives in a theme of failure and hopelessness. Or perhaps they listen to Nancy who hides from the world in a fear-filled theme of her own life.

These therapists sincerely want to help their clients but often find that, despite their clients' pleas for help, there often appears to be a barrier that keeps clients frozen in place and unable to move forward. In some cases it appears that clients even resist therapists' efforts to create change and improvement in their lives.

Clients seek psychotherapy when they feel that they are unable to deal effectively with the changes taking place in their lives. These changes could be in their relationships with others or in their relationships with themselves. Some common catalysts for seeking the help of a therapist range from such complaints as depression, anxiety, parenting, and addictions, to grief and loss. The clients hope the therapist will supply them with the solutions to the problems of living which the clients are encountering and also enduring.

When clients begin therapy, they share their stories with their therapists. These stories usually are embedded within "themes" which the clients have developed about their problems, and these themes can often encompass their entire outlook on life. Themes are created as a way for clients to comprehend and to explain to themselves, as well as to others, their inner experiences of certain situations and events. These themes can also lead to entrenched worldviews which may keep clients locked in a distressing relationship with their problems.

In psychotherapy, the premise of working with clients' themes is that our worldviews are generally self-constructed. Even though there are fundamental facts to be found in the stories of our experiences, most of our stories are simply constructions that we have built, but we often believe that they are factual and unshakable. These concrete constructions create the erroneous belief that our self-manufactured worldviews are factual rather than views that have been created by our own perceptions. When we think that the limited stories we have created are the only stories available, it is no wonder that we feel such angst when life inevitably changes.

Our worldviews are constructed by sets of repeated assumptions that we make. The most basic action of creating an assumption is the drawing of a distinction. The act of drawing a distinction allows the observers to acquire information and comment on their perception of the world. If an observer does not made a distinction, everything would appear to be an indistinguishable mass. For example, distinctions can be drawn along the membrane of an amoeba, separating the inside from the outside, or between the parts of an automobile, placing those parts in specific areas. Our basic ability to understand comes from making distinctions because the drawing of a distinction separates an object from the indistinguishable mass and gives it form. When this separation happens, a boundary is indicated which is then followed by a description from the observer. This action of creating a distinction and then setting a boundary leads to the creation of patterns of separation which the observer repeatedly activates. It is this fundamental process which creates a reality for the one who is drawing the initial distinction (Keeney, 1983).

This drawing of a distinction should not be confused for true reality because "The world we experience as human beings is only one possible way of approaching reality among the infinite other possible systems of distinction" (Neuman, 2003, p. 89). As Spencer-Brown (1969) points out,

> A distinction (something) is drawn by arranging a boundary with separate sides that a point on one side cannot reach the other side without crossing the boundary … Once a distinction is drawn, the spaces, states, or contents on each side of the boundary, being distinct, can be indicated. (p. 1)

The action of drawing distinctions changes the process of describing an experience. Our attempts to describe what has been constructed involves making yet another distinction about the initial distinction. This repetition of making distinctions about distinctions leads to habitual patterns of both perception and behavior which then in turn create higher-order meanings (Keeney, 1983). When we continually repeat these patterns, we begin to believe the patterns and their associated meanings are the true reality and that is just how life really is, we say, unaware that our initial action of drawing distinctions starts a process of reality construction.

These drawing of distinctions and subsequent representations directly affects the biology of cognition. Pulling from the work of noted Chilean biologist Humberto Maturana, Krippendorff (1984) points out,

> The mammalian retina consists of numerous light-sensitive cones, each of which distinguishes magnitudes but no pattern. Information about these magnitudes is not transmitted directly to the brain because, immediately behind the retina, a network of neurons computes relations in the form of differences between

the impulses originating in neighboring cones. Following the first layer of neurons is another one, which now computes differences of differences, which are again transmitted to another layer of neurons, etc. Thus, higher-order patterns are created and information about them ultimately reaches the brain, where it leads to further computations of relations and ultimately of actions that effect a change in the very image that gave rise to the original sensation. Cognition—the sequence of drawing distinctions and computing relations—is in fact circular, involving the observer's nervous system as well as the causal network of the environment. In not insignificant ways, cognition is a function of the biological organization of the observer. (p. 26)

Our use of language is the tool we use to establish our distinctions on the world. Our language separates the world into representations of objects and different categories of objects, while describing ways in which those differing objects can be related. The initial drawing of a distinction leads to the creation of a dichotomy which causes a loss of awareness that there can be other ways by which one can represent events. Our lack of awareness that our knowledge about the world is mediated by our representations of the world cause us to act as if the representations are objective truth instead of subjective constructions of reality.

For us to create meaning from our distinctions we have to separate an "it" from what is "not." We then associate the "it" from what "it is not" with something else. This process of separation is supported by our use of language. Our perceptions are built on the relationship between "it" and "not it." An observer can only experience something as being different from some other thing when it is placed in relation to something else. As Bateson (1972) asserted, it is the differences that we perceive. The ability to perceive an emotion or a behavior rests on the drawing of distinctions by an observer whose distinctions then create a separation from what it is not, which then leads to a relationship between the differences held in place by our language.

These separations are also acts of connection because the boundary that separates also connects that which it separates. As Flemons (2002) states, "Mindful (perceptual and language) acts of separation connect, and thus we will always find ourselves experientially connected to that from which we purposefully separate" (p. 9). This simultaneous act of separation and connection can be problematic when clients want to eliminate a symptom that they regard as their problem. Flemons (2002) reminds us that, "Most clients want you to help them negate their symptom. But given the relational structure of language and thought, any effort in this direction risks further entrenching the very thing they so desperately want eradicated" (p. 12).

Even though no one observation holds the truth about a representation, different observers can mutually corroborate the distinctions that the other has drawn. If different observers' are in agreement about the initial distinction and subsequent representations, this can create a consensus agreement about what is to be considered reality. If we are unaware that it is we who are creating the representations and meanings, then self-fulfilling prophecies and self-reflexive reinforcement of the original distinctions drawn can occur. The self-created reality of the observers will be continually maintained until new distinctions have been drawn. Therapists must gather sufficient information so that they can determine how the clients' distinctions are being created before simply accepting the distinctions that the clients bring (Keeney, 1983).

It is difficult for us to believe that events have no characteristics. Korzybski (1958) asserted that our perceptions of reality are really based on neurological processes that take place on the nonverbal and the verbal levels of experience. When an event takes place, we receive information through our five senses. This information is then sorted and selected by our nervous system, therefore the information we consciously receive already has been abstracted by our nervous system and is only a small part of the original information. From these piecemeal sensations, our nervous system attempts to construct a conscious awareness of the event by matching corresponding patterns of sensory material with our brain's archived record of previous similar experiences.

The initial sensory information is then additionally abstracted and changed as our brains distinguish and associate the information with a specific symbolic representation in the form of a "word." This word is then used to describe the experience of the event. From this level of description, the process continues as we draw inferences and assumptions of the event based on the descriptions we have made. These inferences are then generalized with other experiences we have had in the past.

Our continuing inferences and evaluations of earlier distinctions create higher levels of experience.

Our problems arise when we don't realize that we are the ones who are indeed projecting our experiences onto the event as if it were independent of our abstracting. Humans are the only species that appears to operate on meanings rather than simply responding to primary sensory experience. Animals cease abstracting at the nonverbal level, whereas humans can continue to move to a verbal level of the abstracting process. Not only can we humans abstract beyond the nonverbal level, but we can also make inferences about that which we have abstracted and represent it in symbolic form which takes on meanings.

Suppose one person slaps another person. The first level of description about the event would be something like, "He hit me!" The next level of inference based upon the description could be, "He hit me because he is angry." The next level inference about the last inference could be, "He hit me because he is angry because he didn't like what I said." The next inference about the previous inferences could be, "He hit me because he was angry about what I said and that means that what I said was bad." This process can continue until we reach higher orders. These can generate themes through which the person who was hit may live his life. These themes could be: "What I think and say are never good"; "It is dangerous to speak one's mind"; or "I am a worthless person because of what I think and say." Our responses to events are often taken from higher-order meanings we have created, and these responses often become automatic and reactive. These higher-order meanings then become the themes by which we live our lives.

The initial sensory representations that we experience create schemas, which are collections of ideas. These ideas assist us in organizing those sensory representations with similar attributes. This can be useful since it allows efficient thought about situations or objects. These schemas are then used to group similar situations and objects into categories. For example, the category of "classical music instruments" would contain musical instruments such as trumpets, violins, and cellos, but probably would not contain electric guitars because "classical music" rarely includes this instrument.

After the initial lower levels of descriptions are made and the schemas are developed, then higher-order levels are built, but these higher-order levels leave out some characteristics of the initial sensory experiences. It is the ignoring of most of the characteristics that are specific to any particular event that can move one to the higher orders of abstraction. By abstracting only similar characteristics or schemas, we build "categories" of events. These categories are mental formations, and they do not exist in the natural world. These categories are simply created *by* our inferences *about* our inferences. These categories are what connect objects because they have mutually common characteristics. To comprehend "something," we have to place it within a category which has similar characteristics to other "things."

The classifications of these categories within a set of circumstances (a particular event or series of situations) form a context This context determines the higher meaning of those categories which then leads to encompassing themes which guide individuals' perceptions and reactions to similar descriptions. These constructed contexts are changed either when a category is reclassified as something else or when entirely new objects are introduced into the category. Due to the change in the labeling of the category or new objects placed into the category, the perception of the parts of the category has to change.

Themes are the experiential context in which activity occurs. Context determines the perception and the subsequent reaction that people have to an event. One event can be evaluated in multiple ways by multiple people based on the context in which the event occurs. For example, an angry interaction between a parent and a male adolescent could be perceived as: (1) the normal growing pains of teenagers, (2) parental domination of a child's free spirit, or (3) a rude young man who wants to embarrass his parent. The perceptual outcome will depend on the context into which the argument is placed by the observer. As Bateson (1979) stated,

> Without context, words and actions have no meaning at all. This is true not only of human communication in words, but also of all communication whatsoever, of all mental process, of all mind, including that which tells the sea anemone how to grow and the amoeba what he should do next. (p. 13)

In time, these contexts can become themes which can be either resourceful or dysfunctional.

If we were to see the challenges that our clients bring to therapy as literary themes, we would then have a more flexible overview of the clients' situations. It also keeps therapists from getting stalled and stuck in superficial information which does not actually contribute to change. It is also easier to change the clients' higher-order limiting themes without spending excessive time in problem investigation and lower-level pathology-focused interventions. For example, many therapists have watched themes play out in their offices such as "The Wife Who Can't Trust," "The Man Who Is Angry," "The Frightened Child," or "The Family That Cannot Communicate." These themes are very prevalent in therapy sessions, and as long as therapy is bound up in those themes, any action, discussion, or directive that is produced within that theme will be a component of that very theme (Keeney et al., 2015). Placing too much emphasis on how the theme was created or on who is involved in the theme does little to change the theme.

For example, I worked with a young woman named Allison who sought help in navigating through relationship issues. She told me that no matter who she dated, she found that the man lost interest early in the relationship; he dragged out their eventual breakup. This distressed Allison because she felt powerless to keep it from happening again and again. A theme emerged in the session. She was "The Long Breakup Girl." She had been approaching her relationships from this perspective, and this made her hesitant to fully commit to partners (which is also why her partners eventually pulled away). As long as she starred in the theme of "The Long Breakup Girl," she was setting herself up for more disappointment.

In order to help our clients with their limiting themes, we must change the theme itself. It is necessary to move the therapy out of a theme centered in problems and pathology, and instead move it into new themes of potential and possibility. Since themes hold all the actions and the characters of our clients' stories, their healing and transformation depend on our ability to create a totally different theme that focuses on the clients' resources instead of on their deficits and problems.

By shifting the clinical focus from the problems to the larger themes, therapists can become more flexible in how they work with their clients. Our ability to adjust themes is dependent upon (a) what themes are initially brought to therapy, and (b) what resources each client has available to build new themes. As Papp and Imber-Black (1996) state, "Just as themes enable interviewing possibilities and a new organization of vast amounts of seemingly disconnected material, so do themes facilitate a wide variety of intervention possibilities that are not limited by one method or approach to therapy" (p. 14).

We are not aware that the themes which we build will continue to solidify themselves. Our experiences of an event lead to descriptions of the event, which leads to inferences about the descriptions of the event, which leads to inferences about previous inferences. This creates a continuing spiral which reinforces our higher-order meanings which are based on feedback from the original inferences. These higher levels of abstraction continue due to the circularity of the abstracting process. This recursive process results in a closed system in which higher-order levels feed back into our primary descriptions. This provides us with information that we really believe is about the event, but in reality, it is making the event conform to the higher-order meanings we have created. As Carvalho (2015) states,

> Recursion ... means that not only the result but also the distinction(s) that produced it, constitute the grounding of the next operation of a system. The circularity here implied, as in a self-pointing arrow, can only acquire meaning in its "infinite in finite guise" with the presence of an observer that identifies the sequences of a form that re-enters itself. (p. 3)

If therapists become aware of this circular feedback rather than strictly focusing on the lower levels of experience from a linear cause-and-effect perspective, they can gain more freedom to exercise creativity in shifting contextual themes. Limiting oneself to calculated prearranged therapy interventions instead of focusing attention on higher-order contexts can lock therapists into rigid ways of responding that do not take into consideration the complexity. In fact, the ignoring of higher-order complexity and the placing of excessive attention on eradicating lower-order thoughts, feelings, and behaviors put therapists in a dichotomous fight in which one side has to eliminate the other. Essentially, a linear method is often difficult when working with higher-order complexity.

Changing the higher-order of context/themes creates new perceptions that can then provide feedback to the lower levels which acquire meaning from the feedback. When the theme of a therapy session is changed, the meanings of the lower-level experiences and behaviors changes. Attempted interventions that do not take into consideration higher themes only serve to perpetuate the initial distinctions and subsequent abstractions made by clients about their problems.

Our perceptions of who we are and what we do are based primarily on these higher orders of experience (meaning) and not the lower-order sensory experiences. If this is the case, can we ever really know a true reality that exists outside of the lower-level sensory experiences? It begs the question whether we can ever really know our "self" if we can only ever know the self that is based on our own constructed higher orders of experience. Since we all have had a limited number of events in our lives, it is difficult to ascertain what our self truly is without creating higher-order inferences about those events.

Even though the lower levels of experience may be more subject to change given their contact with the sensory world, the higher-order abstractions are more static because of their assigned symbolic meanings. These limited meanings continue to be categorized as real events or things since their descriptions have not been changed. We often do not realize that our descriptions of experiences are really all metaphorical since the categories have been created by us. Our meanings and metaphors are created to describe nonverbal sensory experiences as a way for us to comprehend and create objective experiences. We forget that our so-called objective reality is really just a metaphor for subjective experiences at the nonverbal level.

As therapists, we should remember that our therapeutic interventions and perspectives are only one way to view client problems. If we continue working inside the problem-oriented themes, we perpetuate the problem. We must make new distinctions about the initial problem. As Papp and Imber-Black (1996) remind us, "When a therapist keeps defining a problem in a way that leads to more of the same, it is a signal to develop a new perspective" (p. 17).

To reiterate, when an event occurs, we have a sensory experience. We will then formulate a description of the event. After that, we will make inferences drawn from our original descriptions. We will then make further inferences about our initial inferences. These inferences are higher-order classifications to which we assign meanings constructed by our language. When we are rigid in our descriptive language, we often become stuck in our theme. When we change our language, then there can be change in our meaning, which then causes a shift in the theme. These new themes take place at the higher orders of our experience which then change lower-level descriptions and inferences. When clients are stuck in limiting higher orders of experience, adjustments to lower levels are often difficult. As Papp and Imber-Black (1996) state, "Since themes address multiple levels of experience, it should come as no surprise that altering a central theme generates a process of change with widening effects in a fairly short period of time" (p. 19).

Thematic contexts can either strengthen or dissolve higher-order experiences. This can occur if the experience category changes or the information inside the category changes. From this perspective, the therapist's main job is not to delve extensively in etiological concerns or battle lower-level dichotomies, but rather help cocreating new themes. Clients can then access their own resources for change to generate healing. This can be counterintuitive for therapists whose training has been primarily centered on lower-level linear interventions that do not take into consideration the larger themes.

There is a dilemma when both therapists and clients are working within the theme that the clients brought to therapy. Resolution of clients' suffering can be hampered if the interventions remain with the same problem-oriented theme. Staying within the same theme locks therapists into trying to find solutions for the problem which only solidify the clients' themes. The interventions at lower levels of experience can maintain the theme which contains all the distinctions that created the theme itself. Therapists may unknowingly be contributing to the perpetuation of the very problem from which clients want to escape. As Keeney et al. (2015) state, "Sometimes therapists are taught to keep clients inside pathological or problem themed contexts because their model needs that framing to be able to conduct its operations. Stated differently, a problem-focused therapist needs a problem in order to perform problem-solving" (p. 40).

The consistent focus on themes related to pathology prevents clients from accessing the empowering resources which could help them transcend their problems. This is because the resources they require are not located inside limiting pathology-laden themes. Regrettably, many psychotherapy interventions only work if both the therapists and the clients stay inside the pathology-focused themes. Most psychotherapists are taught to view the theme that clients bring as problems and then the work is done only within that theme. As they work within a theme that has been labeled as a "problem," therapists see any thought, emotion, or action that occurs inside the theme as a problem.

Therapists often find that predetermined theoretical or technical knowledge may be inadequate in working at the higher levels because of the unique nature of each client's theme. Using standardized, predetermined therapy applications geared toward intervening at lower-level experiences without consideration of the uniqueness of clients' higher-order meanings, therapists may find that they are unable to easily access clients' closed systems of information. The higher orders of experience will continue to feed the lower levels which will perpetuate and help maintain the higher levels. The creation of new higher-order themes will alter "the viewing and the doing" of lower levels because a new higher level of information feeds back to those lower levels (O'Hanlon & Wilk, 1987). These closed systems are more easily accessed when benevolent, favorable themes are introduced.

Exiting from dysfunctional themes requires a change in how clients perceive their initial dysfunctional frames or a shift away from any elements of the problem-oriented theme. Ray and Keeney (1993) use the analogy of a three-act play for helping clients move out of limiting contexts. They see the initial problem as Act One of the therapy session where there is discussion about the "problem" and why it is considered a problem. Act Two is a link to any actions, thoughts, or behaviors which can lead clients away from the problematic context in Act One. Act Three is the final act in which clients experience resolution from the problem found in Act One.

To change higher-order themes in therapy will necessitate an avoiding of a pathology-oriented focus. Continued discussion of the themes of limitation, diagnosing pathology, and emphasizing client deficits are counterproductive. To shift out of the limiting themes, therapists must look for any potential positive client strength or resource in order to construct new themes. This will require a letting-go of prearranged ways of interacting with clients. Because themes are "embedded in a different form of logic, they are capable of releasing the therapist from conventional and redundant ways of thinking" (Papp & Imber-Black, 1996, p. 17).

New empowering or healing themes can be created spontaneously by using information obtained from the client. To discover new themes, the therapist will start wherever the client begins. Then conversation is directed so client distinctions and subsequent themes become more obvious. Therapists must listen intently to the clients' descriptions of their problems as they find larger confining meanings that have been created which block problem-solving or accessing their inner healer. Off-the-cuff remarks or questions about unrelated topics can be used to find exit points from the initial disempowering theme. Therapists are then to observe clients' responses as feedback in order to determine if an attempt to introduce a new theme has resonated with clients. Since there are a plethora of possible distinctions that can be drawn, the therapist is not locked into any one specific theme.

Therapeutic interventions will become more like improvised conversations rather than preset dialoguing. Random comments and observations from the therapist will be needed in order to move out of the initial themes of dysfunction. It is these conversations that offer openings that can lead clients into new possibilities and more empowering themes. The client's problems will not be observed through the linear medical models, but instead they will be seen as a distressed theme. This way of evaluating cases changes the focus of the therapy from lower-order pathology to the higher-order of meaning construction. Therapeutic possibilities are increased since therapist and client are not bound by inflexible cause and effect interventions.

One significant case that impressed upon me the need to focus on larger themes in therapy was the case with which we began this chapter. Maggie and Anthony had come looking for help in dealing with the suicide of their adult son, Michael. When I first met Maggie and Anthony in the office waiting area, I had noticed that they appeared slightly disoriented. Maggie was courteous, but she also appeared to be very stoic. Anthony seemed to be a kind, gentle man who had one of the saddest smiles I had ever seen.

As soon as the session started, both parents began to weep intensely. Maggie informed me that her son had not only committed suicide two weeks earlier, but had done it in front of them. Michael had apparently had a history of mental illness which would come and go with little forewarning of when his next episode would take place. Most of the time, Michael was fine, held a job, and provided for his family. Other times, Michael could act incredibly erratic and become violent; these episodes had increased over the last six months.

Maggie described how she and her husband had gone to visit Michael and found that he was physically attacking his spouse and children. They both rushed to restrain Michael and to protect his family. Maggie then quickly removed Michael's family from the home. When she went back inside to check on Anthony and Michael, Michael ran to a room in the back of the house and returned holding a handgun. Both Maggie and Anthony initially believed that Michael was going to go outside to shoot his family, but instead Michael put the handgun in his mouth and quickly pulled the trigger. Maggie and Anthony both witnessed his suicide and tried desperately to save his life. However, Michael died within a few moments. Maggie's body shook as she described how the life flew out of him as he lay in her arms.

Understandably, this horrific event had emotionally devastated Maggie and Anthony. I wondered to myself if their strong emotional show of grief in the office might have been one of the few instances they had actually allowed themselves to feel the intensity of what occurred. Both parents struggled to talk about what had happened, but after a couple of minutes of trying to talk while sobbing, I told them to not worry about talking and just to allow their emotions to come out. It would be an understatement to describe these parents as emotionally distressed, and to this day I have rarely seen expressions of grief and loss that were as intense.

After ample time was given to them to express their emotions, I expressed my sympathies for what they had been through. They told me how Michael could be such a wonderful son when he was not dealing with his mental health challenges, but they both said they could not get the image of him with the gun out of their minds. Neither had slept much since the incident, and they both said that they were leaning on each other for support. Anthony insisted that if only they could have arrived a few minutes earlier, the situation could have been stopped. He then began sobbing uncontrollably and collapsed back onto the couch and into his wife's arms. I noticed that Maggie cradled him as if he were a scared child needing shelter from the things that terrified him. Maggie began to stare into the distance as she held Anthony.

"He just wasn't in his right mind," Maggie stated. "Yes, he would never had done that if he was his usual self," Anthony said. "He never would have hurt anyone when he was well. He wouldn't hurt a fly when he was not having his problem," Maggie added. "Michael never would have hurt his family when he was not out of his mind. He loved them. He would just lose touch with reality sometimes, and no one could talk to him. He would sometimes get violent. He never did that when he was well," Anthony said. Both began to cry again.

As I sat and listened to these devastated parents, I saw a theme emerging. The theme that came to me was "The Parents Who Saw Too Much." I believed that as long as therapy remained focused on that theme, these two distraught individuals would be trapped in a problem that no one could ever solve. In these kinds of situations, there are no solutions.

Anthony cleared his throat loudly and told me, "It's just that we don't know how to move on after this. Sometimes I catch myself thinking he is still alive. I feel like we can't wake up from this bad dream we are having. I find myself still expecting him to call me. I know that he can't, but I still wish he could." Maggie nodded as Anthony spoke. "I still have his photo on my phone," she said as she showed me Michael's photo. "Every day around 5:30 in the afternoon we both just break down because that is the time he killed himself … the only thing we can do is pray." Maggie's voice trailed off.

When I heard the comment about praying, I asked if Maggie and Anthony were religious. They both said they were very religious and said they believed it was God who helped them get through their days and deal with their grief. They also told me that some of the people they knew had said to them that they should be mad at God for what happened. Anthony stated with a degree of authority in his voice that Michael's suicide was not the fault of God, and neither he nor Maggie placed any blame on anyone or anything. It was a terrible tragedy resulting from Michael's "brain issues." Both he and Maggie agreed that as difficult as things were for them, they could not have dealt with any of the situation without God.

I began to understand that Maggie's and Anthony's faith was a very strong resource that they could access. I asked them if they said prayers during that 5:30 pm time period. They said they did. I then asked if the prayers were spoken aloud, and Maggie said yes and that Anthony was the one who said the prayers. I asked Anthony if he would say a prayer to help us find our way in the therapy session. He sheepishly smiled and nodded yes. Anthony then, with much passion in his voice, said a short prayer in which he asked God for strength and the acceptance to move forward in their lives.

When he had finished, I complimented Anthony on the power and authority he demonstrated in saying his prayer, and he received my compliments well. I then asked if he had ever thought of becoming a preacher. At that moment, both Maggie and Anthony looked surprised and glanced at each other. They both began to cry. "He has always wanted to be a preacher, but he doesn't believe he can do it," Maggie said. Anthony agreed with her, saying that he did want to share "God's word" with others, but he was hesitant. I asked him why he was so hesitant when it was obvious to me that he had a wonderful gift and that it was important to share that gift with others who felt the same way as him.

Anthony insisted that he never thought there was anything special about him. He told me that when he heard other impressive preachers speak, he believed that they seemed to have a special calling that he did not possess. I then asked Anthony if perhaps this terrible tragedy with Michael could be his calling. Maggie and Anthony both appeared to be puzzled by my comment.

I said that unfortunately there are many people in the world who have gone through similar tragedies. I suggested that what makes their own situation different is that they have been through this tragedy, yet they still love God, and desire to share his message. I conjectured that this could be a gift to others who are also grieving from loss. I smiled at Anthony and told him, "Perhaps your calling is hidden in this tragedy."

Anthony and Maggie now appeared to have shifted their mood and were listening closely to what I said. Anthony smiled and told me how much he had always wanted to share the Gospel with other people. He told me that he was just afraid that few people would actually take him seriously. I immediately countered with the assertion that he is a man who has been through one of the worst things that can ever happen and yet he still loves God. "Anthony," I said with a smile, "if people don't take that seriously, then I don't know if they can take anything seriously."

Both Maggie and Anthony began to smile. The energy in the room suddenly shifted from despair to curiosity. I wondered out loud if perhaps they both had a remarkable message to share with others. I told them that it was incredible that with all they had gone through, they both still did not blame God and wanted to share the Gospel with other people. Their level of religious devotion was something that few people get to witness.

Anthony acknowledged what I had said, but countered that he was reluctant to pursue preaching because he wanted to be sure that he was doing it for the right reason. At that moment, the theme of therapy was shifting from "The Parents Who Saw Too Much" to the new theme of "The Reluctant Preacher." This was a theme which held powerful resources which Maggie and Anthony could draw from to work through their grief.

"Anthony," I said, "I am impressed with your humility. There are probably many people who want to become preachers because they want fame, money, or power, but you are a 'reluctant preacher.' You want to preach only for the right reasons. I find that level of dedication and self-awareness inspiring and profoundly spiritual." Maggie agreed, saying that Anthony was very humble and spiritual and that he would do a wonderful job if he decided to become a preacher. I noticed Anthony was sitting up straighter and looked more focused on what was being said. He was unconsciously nodding his head as I spoke.

I told Maggie and Anthony that for the next week, I wanted them to do something very special. They should buy a large, white candle and gather with any other family members who were available every day around 5:30 pm. I wanted them to light the candle and have Anthony say some special healing prayers with a different prayer for every day of the week. I told them that it was very important that healing prayers would be said for all the individuals who were involved in this tragedy. Anthony should include prayers asking for strength and also for direction in pursuing a mission to share their story and to help others. Anthony did not resist this directive. He and Maggie both nodded their head in strong acceptance of what I had asked them to do.

I saw Maggie and Anthony again two weeks later. They both described how they had followed the directive to light a large, white candle and have Anthony pray a healing prayer every day for a week at 5:30 pm. It turned out that different family members and friends also took part in their special ceremonies. They decided to change the time of their ceremonies to 6:30 pm for those who wished to take part but worked until 6 pm. Anthony then excitedly said that after the first week, there had been an increase in the number of people who wanted to attend, and there had been a request to include other topics of loss. Maggie and Anthony had then decided that they would begin to host a weekly gathering in their home to discuss how to apply one's love of God in difficult times. They mutually decided that they would call this once a week gathering "Michael's Hour" in memory of their son.

Maggie now appeared much less stoic, and Anthony showed more signs of confidence in the interaction. Anthony remarked that even though he still did not believe he would be a great preacher, he would have to trust God who would know better than he. Their grief for the loss of their son was not as intense as it had been in our previous session, and Maggie said that she felt there was a renewed sense of partnership with her husband. Anthony said that he was becoming more comfortable with speaking about religious topics, as well as feeling his own emotions. Maggie remarked that she felt inspired by Anthony's prayers and his attempts to share God's love with others. In time, Anthony gained more confidence in preaching to small groups of people, and he and Maggie grew their circle of emotional support through their weekly meetings.

Their journey of healing began as a result of exiting the theme of "Parents Who Saw Too Much." It was when Maggie and Anthony embraced a new theme of Anthony being a "Reluctant Preacher" that they were able to start accessing the resources they needed to move forward. The changing of the theme was not the result of any preplanned intervention, but it emerged spontaneously through the interaction between the three of us.

* * *

When changing themes in therapy, the goal is not to find new solutions, dispute irrational thoughts, or create new narratives about the problem. Instead we seek to generate a new way of relating to what was once considered un-relatable. When the relationship between the clients and what they once perceived as un-relatable changes, it unleashes their potential for creative self-healing. When therapy is centered only on a medical model, pathology-oriented discourse, or the initial themes brought to therapy, any attempted change within those themes can be extremely difficult.

CHAPTER 2

Psychotherapy as theme creation

In the previous chapter, we covered how clients' distinctions construct the meanings of events which in turn can then form into themes which then direct their lives. Our distinctions are solidified by our language which leads to the creation of our explanatory meanings which then in turn lead to overarching themes. These themes are defined within relationships which are defined within larger interactional patterns. To maintain these themes requires a repetitive process of reproducing the meaning in a shared reality. However, the reproduction of these meanings can be altered through experiential interactions with therapists that shift clients' previous perceptions and meanings. When previous meanings shift, and new themes emerge, former interactions and reactions identified as the "problem" then will have to adjust.

An issue in therapy that can arise is when therapists become lost in their clients' own themes. Therapists are then unaware that the same theme is continually replayed throughout the therapeutic interaction. It then does not matter what takes place in the session if the theme being discussed is the same problem-oriented theme the client arrived with. If the problem-oriented theme is not discarded, it will become entrenched in the minds of both the therapist and the client. Continuing in the same theme will only reinforce the initial distinction made by the client. The theme becomes the "thing" that has to be battled and defeated in order for healing to occur.

The reduction of the initial theme to an explainable etiology only continues to focus more attention and more energy on that problematic theme. This unfortunately solidifies the clients' initial perception that there is only one way to view their problem. Regardless of any type of intervention, if both the client and the therapist are unable (or unwilling) to abandon the problematic theme, then there is no other way to view the client's situation as anything but a problem.

The dichotomous perception of "problem/no problem" locks therapeutic dialogue into repeated attempts to be rid of something which can never be fully destroyed. The "problem" is locked into an unending duality with "no problem" cast within that problem-oriented theme. Remember, separations are also acts of connection because the boundary that separates also connects. Doing more and more inside a problem-oriented theme only focuses more and more on the "problem/no problem" dichotomy.

By moving out of problem-oriented themes and into themes which emphasize the clients' resources, the focus can shift away from binary problem-solving. No longer is attention given to therapeutic battle tactics which attempt to overcome undesired cognitions, emotions, and behaviors. Instead, any thought, any feeling, or any action within a new theme of client resourcefulness can move clients into other perspectives on life's trials and tribulations. New perspectives and new meaning emerge from actions and interactions based upon new distinctions formed in the therapy session. Healing comes when connections from the clients' initial problem-oriented themes are bridged to resource-oriented themes. Clients have new ways to relate to their initial problem.

I assert that psychotherapy is itself nothing more than the creation and maintenance of themes. Therapists who operate out of set, standardized methods will often impose a certain theme onto their clients. These predetermined therapy themes can interpret any client action as a validation or explanation for the imposed theme. This will create an endless loop in which discussion centers on the problem, and any attempts to deviate is perceived as actively resisting the therapist's model.

One's reality often depends upon how the observer observes it. How it is observed depends on our interactions and relationships. Proponents of the varying views of pathology and treatment believe their methods are perfectly valid since they share distinctions with others with similar views. From a social constructionist perspective, there is nothing that is real unless there is an agreed-upon consensus among those involved in a form of a relationship. As Gergen (2009) states, "The realities we live in are outcomes of the conversations in which we are engaged" (p. 4). This calls the field of psychotherapy into question because, if reality is an outcome of conversations, one wonders if psychotherapy could ever be rooted in the realm of objective facts. We, as therapists, believe that by studying our clients intently and objectively, we can somehow treat and eradicate symptoms. We forget that we regularly treat these symptoms independently of context or social interactions. We also mistakenly believe that our theories and techniques are objective knowledge instead of constructed distinctions that the field has created.

If therapeutic theories are constructed distinctions made by group consensus, then this challenges psychotherapy's claim of objectivity and its ability to predict and control emotions, thoughts, and behaviors. Objectivity is difficult because observers use their own perceptions to describe what is being observed and "anything said is said by an observer" (Von Foerster, 2003, p. 283). The language which the observer uses to describe the experience is not the experience it represents. As Korzybski (1958) famously stated, "the map is not the territory" (restated by the great Eastern philosophical scholar Alan Watts as "the menu is not the meal"). From Korzybski's viewpoint, the maps of reality are not reality. Even if one has the very best map, it will be a flawed measure of reality because maps are only descriptions of that which is represented. Our brains take incoming information from our senses, and we then create maps of what we perceive. Due to the limitations of our senses and the influence of cognitive biases formed during our lives, we often create internal descriptions of the external world with imperfect information. We then construct mental maps to understand those very descriptions. We become so dependent on these descriptions as a gauge of reality that we forget that we created them. The very act of creating these maps leads to a reduction of what we are mapping because we are limited by our senses and cognitive biases in observing any event in its entirety.

The use of language is merely a representation of "something" and it freezes that "something" into what we believe is a real entity. We forget that we are the ones who are assigning the representations. In truth, we can assign any term to any object or action. Our language is tricky because language itself can have multiple meanings for a specific term. For example, "that is one bad piano player," can mean that one is a "good" piano player. The ways in which we approach people and situations are predetermined by what words we use to describe them. If young people have to work with a person over the age of seventy-five, their initial interactions to the elders will depend on whether they label the person as "an old person" or as "a person of great wisdom."

Our language is the process we use to make differences between things. To make sense of something, we have to differentiate it from what it is not. This moves us into the dreaded "either/or" way of understanding the world. We become more limited in how we interact in the world because of our ability to construct limited meaning within an "either/or" frame. It is only by blurring the distinctions we created between "it" and "not it" that we gain more flexibility in adjusting the meanings we have created.

This process happens individually as well as collectively. As Gergen (2009) points out, "Our verbal constructions are glued to our life circumstances. We not only construct together; we also live out the implications of these constructions" (p. 44). Since our conversations are higher-order abstractions which have meanings about inferences, it is difficult to know if what we have labeled as "truth" is only a metaphor representing our experiences. As Bacon (2018) points out, there is a major difference between "fundamental reality," which is the world of the material, and "constructed reality," which are the inferences and interpretations we create about fundamental reality.

For example, every day we all experience the sun. We can all agree on this fact and fundamental reality. However, our explanations of "why" we experience the sun is subjective and constructive. Certainly, we can point to the rotation of the earth which gives the appearance of the sun rising. This is an explanation that works for most of us in Western culture. However, other cultures have created their own explanations of why the sun rises based on their sensory experiences. For some, it is because a specific deity has started the process. For others, it is due to their daily prayers and rituals. No matter what the "objective truth" may be, each group has its own truth which guides its relationship toward the sun. All have made their own distinctions about the "sun process" and therefore live as if that is a fundamental truth. We may disagree with their assessment of the etiology of the appearance of the sun, but it does not negate the fact that their particular meanings are their shared realities.

Imagine that a couple seeks therapy to help their relationship. The explanations and interventions prescribed by therapists solely depend on their point of view, which has been shaped by their education and life experiences. One therapist may tell this couple that they are reenacting old emotional patterns from previous romantic relationships. Another therapist may state that their issues are rooted in early childhood attachments. Yet another therapist may tell the couple that societal expectations and a culture of patriarchy have caused them to have problems relating to each other. A different therapist may see issues in family hierarchies and structure that need to be adjusted. All of these assertions are clearly themes which therapists believe to be true, but are really interpretations based upon their own understandings of others' theoretical constructions.

What we traditionally have been taught and have accepted is that we operate in our world in a construction held together by our language. We have sensory experiences which we then attempt to label with language. It is in placing these experiences into a certain linguistic category that we are able to communicate the category to others who share those same categorical meanings. Gergen (2009) reminds us that, "Understandings of the world are achieved through coordination among persons—negotiations, agreements, comparing views, and so on ... Nothing exists for us as an intelligible world of objects and persons until there are relationships" (p. 6).

These categories of language will often determine how solutions of constructed problems will proceed. Therapists' use of language to explain problems may include such diverse distinctions as "ego," "cognitive distortions," "unconditional positive regard," etc. Each constructed explanation will then lead to constructed solutions that are based on the original distinctions made by the therapist. The terminology for understanding the symptoms will automatically cause the therapist to see the "truth" of their perception of the pathology because of their preconceived understanding built by their shared language. The belief that some therapy language is closer to truth than other therapy language is therefore a flawed notion. A variety of languages constructed by individuals based on their perceptions and meanings were constructed due to their reaction to sensory experiences.

These therapeutic explanations of symptoms "have come to function as truth telling within the rules of a particular game—or more generally, according to certain conversations of certain groups" (Gergen, 2009, p. 10). From this position, we can state that the language used in different psychotherapy theories is constructed, is specific to that particular theory, and cannot fully describe the world as it is. Psychotherapeutic language is a further abstraction away from the initial perception of an event or situation, but because of a consensus between individuals in the psychotherapy field, this language becomes real to those who share the same meanings. It is in these meanings that themes have emerged which have guided therapy applications since the very beginning.

A brief history of psychotherapy themes

Psychotherapy can be defined as a procedure for treating mental health issues that involves talking with a professional who is trained to help people cope with life's challenges. At present, there are hundreds of different theories and techniques used in the practice of psychotherapy, but all of them have in common the goal of mitigating mental and emotional suffering. Even though psychotherapy has been around since the 1880s, from a historical perspective, it is a recent invention because the roots of Western psychological healing can be traced back thousands of years.

About 2,500 years ago, thinkers in Greece wrote about the phenomenon of mental illness and also about ways to alleviate the suffering of those who were afflicted by it. Plato asserted that mental health issues arose when one's soul became imbalanced because its rational and irrational components became separated. His student, Aristotle, believed that mental illness occurred when mysterious vapors emerged from one's heart and built up in the brain which clouded perception. The father of medicine, Hippocrates, believed that dysfunctional mental states were due to malfunctions of the brain. Stoic philosophers believed logical discourse could remedy mental and emotional affliction (Thomason, 2005).

After the fall of the Roman Empire, mental illness was explained and treated through the lens of religion and spiritual perspectives, and illness was attributed to demons, witchcraft, or punishment from God. This view of mental illness remained consistent until the nineteenth century when people who suffered from emotional problems were being labeled as deficient or defective instead of bewitched or possessed. The creation of mental institutions to house these individuals continued the process of moving mental illness away from a spiritual problem to a medical problem as more doctors began to work in such institutions (Thomason, 2005).

Some historians cite the true beginnings of Western psychotherapy as the work of Franz Anton Mesmer (Crabtree, 1993). Mesmer, with whom the term "Mesmerism" originates, was a German physician in the 1700s. He believed that a special fluid circulated through the human body and affected its functioning similar to the magnetic forces which affect the solar system. Mesmer believed that when this magnetic fluid was influenced by an outside practitioner, the inner workings of the human body could be affected. Initially Mesmer believed that the use of magnets with his patients was necessary because this inner fluid was magnetic in nature. Mesmer devised a variety of practices with his magnetic therapy which apparently yielded enough success to make him famous across Europe.

In time, Mesmer abandoned his use of magnets, believing his own body could balance the magnetic forces of a patient's body by his focusing intensely and passing his hands over the patient's body. After this change in procedure, the practice of Mesmerism began to shift its focus more toward the psychological aspects of patients. This change was mostly due to the Marquis de Puységur, a leading student of Mesmer's and a member of the French aristocracy. He began to use the Mesmerism system to treat his patients' mental and emotional states. This may have been a critical change in the history of how psychological issues were treated and made future concepts of psychotherapy more acceptable (Crabtree, 1993). Within a few years, Mesmer's beliefs about magnetic fluid were abandoned when it was determined that it was the use of suggestion and expectancy which made possible Mesmer's and his followers' successful outcomes.

It is usually assumed that the beginning of modern psychotherapy was initiated by the work of Sigmund Freud. There were earlier researchers and practitioners, such as Pierre Janet, who greatly contributed to the field; however, Freud is usually seen as the founder of the first true systematized psychotherapeutic approach. Freud, who was trained as a medical doctor at the University of Vienna, developed a deep interest in the treatment of mental illness. He sought training under a famed French neurologist, Jean-Martin Charcot, in hypnotic interventions for psychopathology. Freud was fascinated with Charcot's assertion that the symptoms of illness which had no organic basis were the result of the patient's earlier traumatic episodes. Charcot believed that the neurotic behavior that some of his patients exhibited was due to their intense experiences endured at very early periods of their lives.

Freud took this perspective into his work with Josef Breuer, a Viennese physiologist who also was fascinated by the dimensions of the human mind. Freud and Breuer eventually released their landmark text, *Studies on Hysteria* (1895d), which details their work with a patient whom they referred to as "Anna O." She suffered from what was referred to at the time as "hysteria," but which today would be diagnosed as "conversion disorder." Breuer claimed to have alleviated Anna O's condition through the use of hypnosis, which allowed her to recall traumatic memories from her past which had been blocked by her conscious mind. Once she was consciously aware of her memories, Breuer reported that her symptoms dissipated.

Freud ultimately combined Charcot's and Breuer's ideas about the unconscious presence of previous trauma and bringing that unconscious information into the realm of the conscious mind. This would produce a cathartic release which could end the emotional unrest. The result was Freud's therapy of psychoanalysis, which became a foundational part of psychology, and also had a tremendous influence on Western culture. Freud's ideas about biological drives, unconscious motivations, and repression of sexuality were both alarming and enthralling to those in the field of psychology and the general public as well. His belief was that what people were actually aware of was only a very small aspect of the human consciousness and this was a fundamental component of psychotherapy for many years. Freud asserted that the unconscious mind was the depository of all of our past experiences and that many of these experiences have been repressed in order to defend us from these unpleasant memories. This idea had an influence on such varied areas as politics, art, and literature (Neuringer, 1992; Rabaté, 2002; Shinebourne, 2006).

As a therapy, psychoanalysis was engaged in a rigorous probing into the workings of the unconscious mind. Freud's use of such techniques as "free association" and "dream analysis" was designed to gain access to his patients' unconscious processes. This access would allow Freud to obtain important hidden information that he could use to free his patients from their emotional turmoil. Freud believed that these problems arose from the repressed sexuality and aggression which was prevalent among his restrained, upper-class Victorian clientele.

In Freud's theories we see the creation of an overarching theme which guided his interventions and explanations. The theme of psychoanalysis can be described as a battle against the dark forces of the unconscious mind. If a client exhibited a symptom, that symptom would immediately be placed within the theme of these unconscious conflicts. A nervous habit instantly became tied to moral or neurotic anxiety. Controlling behavior would become anal-retentive fixations. The initial problems which clients brought to Freud remained the focus of the therapy sessions. The theme of psychoanalysis was centered on the acceptance of the client's themes of distress. Those themes were then relabeled to fit the perspective designated by the therapist's model of understanding. Even though the terminology for the problem changed, the problem distinction remained, and both therapists and clients would battle symptoms from a theme of unconscious limitation and dysfunction.

Despite widespread acceptance of Freud's ideas, there were also reactions against them. Especially controversial was the view that emotional suffering is chiefly embedded in repressed sexuality. Two of Freud's close associates broke with him because of Freud's insistence that behavior is primarily directed by innate sexual drives. Alfred Adler and Carl Jung both found that Freud's unbending devotion to his own theories limited their own psychotherapeutic ideas and discoveries. New psychotherapy themes then began to emerge as these former colleagues pursued their own paths.

Alfred Adler was one of the first of Freud's inner circle to break from the dominant perspectives of psychoanalysis. Adler came to believe that neurotic behavior was due to an individual's sense of inferiority, and emotional suffering was the result of unconscious attempts to overcome these feelings of inferiority. His theory was that an "inferiority complex" drives individuals to gain superiority and also accounts for people's unconscious actions. This idea was in opposition to Freud's insistence that sexual drives are the origin of one's thoughts, emotions, and behaviors. Like Freud, Adler also saw child development as crucial to understanding mental health; however, Alder focused on early developments and social interactions rather than Freud's "psycho-sexual" stages (Adler, 1930).

Adler created new themes in explaining human behavior and motivation, yet his therapy, although more positive in tone than Freud's, was still focused on the client's problematic themes. Despite his shifting away from an emphasis on repressed sexual drives, Adler did continue to use a strict explanatory theme when working with his clients. His clients were no longer fighting the dark forces of the unconscious from the psychoanalytic theme, but now they were all fighting within a theme of inferiority/superiority dynamics. The distinctions that originally moved clients to seek therapy were again supported and relabeled by the therapist into a predetermined problem-oriented theme.

Carl Jung also broke with Freud over the idea that sexual drive is the primary motivation in humans. Jung and Freud also vehemently disagreed over the role of mysticism and Jung's belief in a "collective unconscious." Jung defined this "collective" as a universal form of one's personal unconscious which contains memories and symbols that Jung labeled as "archetypes." Jung believed these archetypes were passed down biologically generation to generation and were themes which expressed familiar cross-cultural experiences. Jung said that the integration of these archetypes in one's life was a major goal for personal growth and mental health (Jung, 1960). Therapeutic techniques, such as active imagination, were used to access unconscious archetypes in his clients. He examined and explored such diverse areas as mythology, alchemy, and astrology to better understand the human psyche.

Jung's mystical-tinged therapy was a major change from Freud's deterministic views of human nature, and his ideas about introversion and extroversion, persona, complexes, and synchronicity became important components of modern psychology. Even though Jung's ideas about psychotherapy were more esoteric than Freud's, he still utilized a predetermined theme for his clients. If a client brought a specific condition, Jung would have accepted that theme and then would have placed his own thematic distinctions upon the client. Instead of Freud's sexual drive impulses being the root of client problems, Jung would see the presence of archetypal-related issues which required archetypal-related technical applications.

A new theme of psychotherapy emerged in the 1920s with the arrival of behaviorism. Behaviorism was a reaction to Freud's ideas as behaviorism proponents said they were unable to measure or to observe the unconscious mind. The absence of any objective measurements compelled such early behaviorists as John B. Watson to focus his attention on the observable actions of clients instead of trying to interpret their actions. Behaviorism rejected the model of psychoanalysis because of its lack of scientific scrutiny and placed the etiology of human behavior exclusively in the areas of learning and conditioning.

Behaviorism dismissed the focus on the clients' past histories and instead directed the focus onto the present where behaviors could be objectively measured and then hopefully adjusted. Watson believed that humans could be changed and trained using a methodical and mechanistic manner because it is their responses to stimuli in their environment that form their behavior (Watson, 2017). The resulting therapies that were associated with behaviorism held that the basis of human behavior is mainly learned. To create change in clients, these behavior-oriented therapies focused on applications such as exposure to certain stimuli and using reward and punishment to alter actions.

Even though behavior therapy was a complete change from the past-oriented/unconscious focused therapies, clients were still placed in a predetermined theme. Client problems were created by conditioning and learned responses. A client's anxiety was no longer unconscious impulses, unresolved inferiority complexes, or archetypal issues, but simply the result of a nervous system that had been conditioned to respond in a certain way. Clients were moved into a preset theme which involved predetermined actions used for change.

The development of humanistic psychology and associated humanistic therapies was a reaction to the deterministic methods of Freud's psychoanalysis and Watson's behaviorism. Instead of seeing their clients as captives of their repressed unconscious drives or robotic entities that only respond to stimuli, humanistic therapies declared that clients possessed free will to make the best choices for themselves if they have a sense of personal worth. Humanistic therapists contended that clients have an innate drive to grow psychologically and to discover meaning and fulfillment. Instead of focusing on unconscious complexes or stimulus-response patterns, humanistic therapy saw more importance in the exploration of clients' sense of self. For such luminaries as Carl Rogers, the heart of therapy was the relationship between the client and the therapist and the establishment of a nonjudgmental environment where clients had the freedom to search their own thoughts, emotions, and actions (Rogers, 1946).

Humanistic therapies created new themes for their clients that were vastly different from previous theories. These therapies added new descriptions to psychotherapy such as Rogers' "unconditional positive regard," Fritz Perls' "organismic holism," James Burgental's "existential search for authenticity," and Abraham Maslow's "self-actualization." These new ideas brought a much more positive and much less pathological tone to psychotherapy. However, it was yet another theme which sought to explain and then overcome the problem distinctions made by clients.

Around the same time as humanistic therapies began their encroachment into the field, the cognitive therapies appeared. In the 1950s, Albert Ellis began to shift the focus of therapy away from past-oriented unconscious related therapies toward a present-centered method that focused on clients' irrational beliefs. Ellis contended that it was not psychodynamic unconscious factors that created problems for clients, but rather it was how clients think about the situations that occur in their lives. For Ellis, faulty thinking caused emotional distress rather than the situation itself. His therapy, rational emotive therapy, emphasized the necessity of teaching clients to investigate and challenge what and how they were thinking (Ellis, 1994).

Similarly, psychiatrist Aaron T. Beck noticed that his clients were often distraught because of their internal dialogue and their subsequent emotions rather than the events that had taken place. Beck discovered that his clients often displayed many errors in their thought processes which contributed to their emotional distress. By attending to the distortions and overgeneralizations in his clients' thinking, Beck discovered that his clients made considerable progress in controlling their own emotions and actions (Beck, 1993).

Different from the behavioral therapies, which regarded cognition as a secondary process that arises during stimulus-response, the theme of cognitive therapies was that the clients' thoughts were of primary importance in ending emotional suffering. The adoption of cognitive-related techniques created a change in how therapy was approached. In time, this theme of cognitive processes as the root of problems evolved as new models emerged which blended the "cognition as etiology" concept with such accompaniments as cognitive-behavioral modification, mindfulness, and mental imagery training.

Presenting an even more significant difference from psychoanalysis and cognitive-behavioral based therapies, was the arrival of family systems therapy. This form of therapy moved attention away from a focus on individuals and placed it more on the interactions which occurred between individuals, specifically members of a family. Clients' problems were no longer seen as the result of individuals' personality and behavior, but were more the result of issues in communication and social relationship patterns.

Family systems therapy grew out of the work of the "Bateson Project" in 1952, a government-funded project to study the communication patterns of schizophrenics, led by anthropologist and cyberneticist, Gregory Bateson. Bateson invited future notable therapy figures, Jay Haley, a graduate student in communication, John Weakland, an anthropologist, and psychiatrists Don Jackson and William Fry, to the group. Within a year of the group's formation, some members of the group also began interacting with Milton Erickson to learn more about Erickson's groundbreaking hypnotic work.

The group began to carefully study the strange and absurd conversational patterns exhibited by schizophrenics. They found that many of these patterns did not make sense unless they were examined within the context of their families. The shift to examining the communication patterns of schizophrenics and their families led the group to advance the idea that schizophrenics often have conflicting messages from family members. The Bateson Project found that these incompatible messages, when connected to an insistence for response, create a context in which the response by the schizophrenic will always be viewed by the family as incorrect. As the group believed there was no escape from the dysfunctional interactional context, the group concluded that the schizophrenic has no alternative response other than with communication patterns which are deemed "crazy."

The group published the landmark study "Toward a Theory of Schizophrenia", in which they stated,

> From this theory and from observations of schizophrenic patients is derived a description, and the necessary conditions for, a situation called the "double bind"—a situation in which no matter what a person does, he "can't win." It is hypothesized that a person caught in the double bind may develop schizophrenic symptoms. (Bateson et al., 1956, p. 251)

This study, although presently dismissed as an answer for the etiology of schizophrenia, did spark a therapeutic movement which shifted the focus away from an interpretation of individuals and more toward a focus on contexts and interaction patterns.

In time, family therapy became influenced by the field of cybernetics, and general systems theory. The view was adopted that the family is a structure which develops homeostatic feedback in order to maintain balance in its functioning. From this perspective, problems brought to therapy are not individual problems rooted in unconsciously repressed drives, but are interactional and relational problems. Attention was paid to the arrangement of family hierarchies, boundaries, and structure. From a relational context, individuals are not pathologized because any problem is seen as part of an interactional pattern of behaviors so no specific individual is to blame. From the family system perspective, the theme of therapy was that, if individuals are showing symptoms of pathology, it is because those individuals are in dysfunctional interactional patterns of a family or social system. Further developments in the family therapy field included emphasis on such concepts as differentiation, attachment styles, and the use of genograms.

As one can see, the development of psychotherapy has resulted in a wide variety of models which all claim to help clients' emotional issues. With the vast amount of development and training in all of these different models, one would assume that there is a clear style or school of thought which produced better outcomes than the others. In spite of the claims of superiority by proponents of therapeutic theories, research has glaringly shown us that there is no particular theory or technique which outperforms the others. In fact, research shows us that it is quite the opposite.

When differing psychotherapeutic approaches were compared, minimal-effect size differences between theories and techniques were discovered. Even though the varying applications are fundamentally different from each other, research has found that all of the major theories and techniques essentially were equally effective. These findings have been called the "dodo bird" effect, named after a character in Lewis Carroll's *Alice in Wonderland*, who, after a race ended stated to the participants, "Everybody has won so all must have prizes." The result of this research empirically showing little difference in effectiveness between therapy approaches has led to an effort to discover the similar factors involved in causing therapeutic change in all of the different psychotherapies. These factors, known as "common factors," are not linked to any one specific model of therapy, but they accentuate the commonality of all the major theories (Duncan et al., 2010; Greenberg, 2016; Wampold, 2015). The common factors include such aspects as therapeutic relationship qualities, therapist qualities, and client expectancies. Wampold and Imel (2015) found that even though psychotherapy is effective, with greater effects than some medical interventions, it is not specific techniques or approaches which obtain better results than others. The role of the therapeutic alliance, which consists of such aspects as empathy, collaboration, goal setting, and expectation, are more strongly related to successful outcomes than specific theories.

A strong therapeutic alliance helps clients to feel cared for and understood; however, in order to have a solid alliance with their clients, therapists must prioritize nonjudgmental listening and acceptance. A strong therapeutic alliance also generally showcases a sensitivity to clients' emotional states, as well as supportive attention when clients describe their experiences. Research has found that the therapeutic alliance has a very substantial impact on the therapeutic change process, and the stronger the therapist–client alliance is, the greater the probability of improvement in client symptoms (Johansen et al., 2013; Priebe et al., 2011).

Wampold and Imel (2015) found that clinical experience does not necessarily make better therapists, and those who adhere strictly to a method do not obtain any better results than those who are more flexible in their approach. It was also found that proponents of a particular treatment who claim that their treatment is effective due to specific elements of those treatments, are not correct. In dismantling studies, when those specific elements were removed, the efficacy of the treatment was not reduced, which suggests those specifics were not the important therapeutic factor in creating change.

What was also surprising was that, in many cases, nonprofessional therapists often performed as well as experienced clinicians. This has cast doubt even on the effectiveness of therapeutic techniques. In a radical landmark study by Strupp and Hadley (1979), the efficacy of professional therapists was compared with the results of college professors who worked with students who were suffering from depression and anxiety. Strupp and Hadley found that, between the college professors and the professional therapists, there were no significant differences in outcomes. These shocking results were a blow to professionals who had come to believe that the specific treatments, as well as the in-depth training on the part of the therapist, led to successful outcomes with clients. Subsequent research has unfortunately shown that Strupp and Hadley's assessment of psychotherapy was accurate. The belief that there is a specific base of knowledge for helping emotional suffering which is only known by psychotherapy professionals is simply not true. This tells us that, despite the many years of intense training, education, and experience required in the field of psychotherapy, it is possible that someone with very little or no training as a professional therapist could be just as successful as a trained and experienced therapist.

The implication of all these studies is that the amount of training, experience, and knowledge of theories has little effect on therapeutic outcomes. This is heresy of the highest order for a field that is built on the belief that training and theories are what create change. This requires a major shift in one's thinking about psychotherapy. As Bacon (2018) states,

> Fully accepting that "techniques lack inherent power" is not simply accepting research results, it means accepting that what masquerade as techniques are an infinite variety of constructed realities limited only by the investment of the client and the creativity and respectability of the therapist. The positive effect is

achieved by the relationship and the process of constructing and deconstructing worldviews; it is not achieved by applying scientific principles to functional reality. (p. 76)

We practitioners are left to contemplate how such a variety of therapies with so many different etiological views could all be so equally effective. The research appears so counterintuitive to what most therapists believe (and are taught) that often those who read these results either refuse to acknowledge the research or operate in a state of willful ignorance. Bacon (2018) believed that to understand the fundamental factor that connects the variety of therapies together it is necessary to adopt the view that psychotherapy functions in a constructed, rather than fundamental, reality. Psychotherapy is a field which does not possess "privileged knowledge" of theories and applications that are essential for specialists in a field to achieve success. Examples of fields that have privileged knowledge are medicine, engineering, and computer science, and all of these fields are based in fundamental reality because they all work in the material world. No matter who in the field performs the application, the results will usually be the same. If a field does not have privileged knowledge, it will function within a constructed reality. In fundamental reality, techniques and training are what create differences in outcomes; the lack of significant effect in techniques or training gives credence to the idea that psychotherapy operates in a constructed reality (Bacon, 2018).

From this evaluation, we see that the successful practice of psychotherapy is not about applying standardized applications. It is about creating a theme to solve the client's problem, on which both the therapist and the client agree. If no one theory or technique is superior to the other, then we cannot say that a particular way of working with clients is the "best." Psychotherapy does work, but it does not seem to work in a way which lends itself easily to cut and dried applications in the way that setting a broken arm would work. It seems that success in a therapy session has more to do with cultivation of the therapeutic relationship and how open and accepting clients are to the particular theories (themes) which therapists supply.

Imagine that a client named Thomas seeks help from a therapist for his depression. The success of the treatment will depend on how comfortable Thomas feels with the therapist and his own acceptance of the therapist's ideas and distinctions. If Thomas seeks help from a psychodynamic therapist, he will participate in insight-oriented exploration of his unconscious mind. If Thomas seeks help from a cognitive behavioral therapist, he will participate in an examination of how his thoughts affect his feelings and actions. If Thomas seeks help from a humanistic therapist, he will evaluate his authenticity, meaning in life, and unconditional positive regard. If Thomas seeks help from a family systems therapist, he will expect to consider other members of his family and to investigate family dynamics, hierarchies, and structures. All of these are completely different themes and, according to outcome research, can work. However, any of these therapeutic orientations will work only if both Thomas and the therapist agree that they will work. If Thomas cannot accept the distinctions and related themes provided by the therapist, then very little success may follow. Just because the therapist believes in the theme he or she is using or because this particular theme has worked with other clients, does not necessarily mean that it will resonate or motivate Thomas.

Effective and transformative therapy is generally not a standardized, regimented process, but rather a dynamic cocreation between the therapist and the client. When therapists realize that their predetermined themes are no better or no worse than any other psychotherapeutic theme, they can let go of allegiance to or reliance on those themes. Therapists can then decide to create new themes in the present moment based on what is actually happening to their clients in real time rather than using a scripted process supplied by those who have never met the client. The history of psychotherapy has been predominantly based on different theoretical factions fighting for dominance in a field which appears to favor none of them. Again, therapists forget that they too are making distinctions in treatments and assessments that are constructed but not founded in fundamental reality. This becomes very obvious in the act of diagnosis.

Diagnosing as theme creation

The view that our perceptions are based on a collective construction can also apply to assertions of psychopathology. The diagnosing of clients is in itself the construction of a theme by the therapist. If the therapist applies a specific label to the client's symptoms, then a theme is automatically constructed which the therapist is now locked in. If a diagnosis of "depression" is given, then the theme of the session will usually be geared toward the depression. This theme can be solidified by the therapist's continued therapeutic applications to rid the client of depression (even though it was the therapist who gave that particular theme to the client). If the client does agree that the theme of "depression" is suitable, both parties will continue to act upon that diagnostic theme for better or for worse. From this perspective theme, the subjective experience of the client has been labeled as something that is "bad" and needs to be removed.

Diagnosing clients with mental health disorders is a subjective construction that is rampant in the field of therapy. It has been reinforced by the need for mental health professionals to obtain payment from third parties, such as insurance companies and government entities. It is common for individuals who enter the field of psychotherapy to be taught that, before any intervention begins, clients must be diagnosed with a predetermined category of disorder. However, from a theme-oriented therapeutic perspective, problems are only problems when someone has labeled them as problems. As Gergen (2009) states, "Problems don't exist in the world as independent facts; rather we construct worlds of good and bad, and define anything standing in the way of achieving what we value as 'a problem'" (p. 4). The more time that is spent in a disorder-related theme, the more likely that particular theme will take root and become reality to both therapist and client. Therapists should be aware that the historical use of the term "diagnosis" suggests the existence of an ailment that in turn requires specific medical actions that focus on treating the ailment. The very act of using a diagnosis can bring a predominant focus and emphasis on pathology thus minimizing the investigation of client strengths and resources.

Therapists usually forget that their own observation of therapeutic interaction is limited to the distinctions that they themselves make. Any distinction the therapist makes, be it an assessment, a diagnosis, or an intervention, is constructed by the therapist. This construction, if accepted by the client, is then cocreated as a reality in the therapy session. As Jay Haley, the founder of strategic family therapy, pointed out,

> When a therapeutic problem is defined as the social relationships of clients, a therapist must include himself in the issue since he helps define the problem. To label a child a "delinquent" or as suffering from "minimal brain dysfunction," or to label an adult as an "alcoholic" or a "schizophrenic," means that one is participating in the creation of a problem in such a way that change may be made more difficult. A therapist who describes a family situation as characterized by "a dominating mother and a passive father" or "a symbiotic relationship between mother and daughter" has created problems, although the therapist might think he is merely identifying the problems put before him. The way one labels a human dilemma can crystallize a problem and make it chronic. (Haley, 1987, p. 2)

The role of diagnosis in psychotherapy has been a source of much dispute over the past fifty years. Despite disagreements about its use, diagnosing has become an important part of the practice of psychotherapy. Having a diagnosis represents the existence and legitimacy of a mental disorder. Often the assigning of a diagnosis will determine the form of treatment that will be applied by the mental health professionals, much in the way a medical doctor would prescribe a course of action for patients. This medicalization of mental health has created the widespread labeling of various social phenomena which has aided sociopolitical forces in determining what is to be considered normal or abnormal. Some have even suggested that the push for diagnosing is due to financial aspirations rather than a desire to create successful therapeutic outcomes. As Horwitz (2011) states, "The research psychiatrists who established the diagnoses were acutely aware of factors such as the need to have diagnoses suitable for obtaining third-party reimbursement, credibility in the broader culture, and dominance over competing mental health professions" (p. 50).

There is also much debate about the role of language in diagnosing. Some believe that the language used in the most recent *Diagnostic and Statistical Manual of Mental Disorders* (DSM) is unreliable. It was found that the extent to which a client was diagnosed with a mental disorder by one practitioner, and would receive the same diagnosis from a different practitioner, was much lower than expected (Chmielewski et al., 2015). It has been argued that the DSM has far too many problems itself which compromise any of its potential benefits. Poland (2015) states, "The categories exhibit substantial heterogeneity, confusing comorbidities, and poorly defined phenotypes, each of which is problematic for research purposes. As a consequence, research has tended to produce findings that are negative, non-replicable, inconsistent, weak, non-specific, or uninterpretable" (p. 25).

Mental health professionals who accept these diagnostic categories overlook the fact that the categories are not inherently real since they too have been constructed. Even the most commonly seen disorders are still distinctions made by a collective group of individuals. For example, even though anxiety disorders comprise one of the more prevalent categories of mental health disorders, there is disagreement in the field whether the assumption that people who suffer from anxiety are indeed experiencing a psychiatric illness. Millions of individuals are diagnosed with various forms of anxiety whose etiology is attributed to such causes as neurochemistry, unresolved childhood issues, or contemporary living in the twenty-first century. In regard to the diagnosing of anxiety, Dowbiggin (2009) states,

> Some observers target the ever-increasing pace and demands of modern life. Nonetheless, a larger body of evidence suggests that the prevalence of anxiety is due less to these pressures themselves than to a prevailing social ethos that teaches people that anxiety-related symptoms are a socially and medically legitimate response to life in the modern age. (p. 429)

I once worked with a woman—I will call her Brenda—who came to see me at the urging of her psychiatrist. The psychiatrist had given Brenda the diagnosis of borderline personality disorder and believed that she needed intensive therapy in addition to her medication treatment. Brenda was very upset by many factors, but one in particular distressed her: the diagnosis. After receiving the diagnosis, Brenda had read about the disorder and became distraught. She could not deny that she had some of the symptoms of the disorder, but she had a hard time with her label. Yet in some ways, she had accepted the label and had already begun to build a new identity around it. Any action was now put inside a theme of borderline personality disorder, no matter how big or how small. She was distressed that she had the diagnosis, and the symptoms of her distress became yet another verifying symptom that solidified her diagnosis. She had become trapped by her diagnosis, and this was not helping her emotional state.

I had already had some experience working with clients who had been labeled as borderline, and something told me that, in spite of some of her symptoms, Brenda was not the "classic" borderline personality that her doctor believed that she was. She certainly had extreme mood swings, could be very explosive and emotionally reactive, had episodes of despair and depression, and exhibited a very poor self-image. In talking with Brenda and finding out a little bit about her past history, it became clear very quickly why Brenda was having so much inner turmoil. Her past was littered with traumatic events which had created a perceived, consistent need for her brain to be on guard, overly controlling, and to overreact emotionally.

Brenda had suffered long-term sexual abuse from her father and uncle which had created a foundation of severe anxiety in her. She had coped the best she could with her situation while she was young. At the first chance, when she was old enough to leave her family, she married the first man who had shown any interest in her. It turned out that he was also physically and sexually abusive. Her few years of being married had made her brain react even more intensely in its efforts to control situations and people so that she could feel safe. She was constantly fearful and that fear emerged as intense and aggressive emotions that wreaked havoc in her relationships.

Since the "borderline" diagnosis clearly was an issue for Brenda, instead I began to reframe her symptoms as efforts to protect herself. I let her know that even though these patterns had a positive intention for her, they were operating on old and outdated emotional programming which needed to be "upgraded." I assured her that even though she had been given a specific diagnosis, that this was only one way to see human behavior. I told Brenda that I knew her doctor's reputation, and it was very good. I told her that the doctor was helping her the best way possible within the doctor's particular way of working with people. However, I worked a little differently, and I would be more interested in her patterns of behavior and less interested in her previous diagnosis. I discussed with her the effects of post-traumatic stress disorder (PTSD) and educated her on how some symptoms of PTSD can seem strange, weird, and even crazy to those who are on the outside looking in. I told her that I needed her help with knowing what was happening with her patterns. I told her that I needed "a Dr. Watson to my Sherlock Holmes" in our sessions because we both wanted to be good detectives to understand how those patterns operated. She agreed to be my partner in our quest to discover the answers to the mystery of her patterns.

From that point on, Brenda and I began our work as "pattern detectives." We cocreated a way of working in which each of us analyzed her reactive patterns to discover how they occurred and what positive intention each pattern had. An example of this detection was a situation in which Brenda became easily frustrated and snapped at her husband. We would then find the original positive intention of the pattern of her snapping when she became frustrated. Usually it was her unconscious desire to change her emotional state and take control of her situation. This way of examining her patterns placed her actions in a new theme of therapy. They were no longer the horrible results of having a personality disorder, but instead they were simply patterns which had the highest intentions of trying to help her feel safer. Brenda discovered that instead of hating these patterns and becoming distraught when they happened, she could begin the long process of making peace with them. This opened the door for her to slowly begin making small adjustments to those patterns. In time, she found that the small adjustments she was making helped her to feel more of the comfort she had been seeking.

Even though Brenda still struggled with her moods and erratic behavior, in time the "pattern detectives" found that Brenda was decreasing the intensity of her outbursts and her emotions. Truthfully, Brenda's emotions could still be intense for most people, but those who knew her began to notice that she was less reactive. I truly believe that if we had continued to operate out of a theme of "borderline personality disorder" instead of making Brenda an active participant in a new "pattern detective" therapeutic theme, I doubt that we would have made much headway in therapy. This shift, from an identity-freezing diagnosis to a less pathological and more participatory role, gave Brenda a feeling of being more in control in her therapy sessions. She became more accepting and accountable for her actions. The hopelessness that she had felt began to disappear.

The variety of disorders in the DSM are in themselves themes which too many psychotherapists have accepted as a real entity. A person diagnosed with borderline personality disorder is thus labeled due to the diagnostic criteria devised by a select group of researchers. There is no inherently borderline personality in nature. The emotions and actions of a person have been labeled as a "thing" which exists apart from the basic level of sensory experience. The lack of irrefutability of the DSM is obvious in how often changes have occurred in the DSM over the past fifty years because new distinctions were made (for example, homosexuality was considered a diagnosable mental disorder until 1975). As Poland (2015) states,

> Given that DSM categories are not associated with specific diagnostic tests and that DSM-based research has not provided well-confirmed specific models and findings concerning the categories, researchers cannot supplement a diagnosis with a consensually validated model of pathology or etiology (although many hypotheses abound). (p. 31)

There appears to be no end in sight to either the use of the DSM or to practitioners' consistent desire to diagnose. Realizing that any diagnosis automatically creates a specific theme that can direct the therapy session should give pause to therapists. Are therapists unwittingly being locked into themes of disempowerment and pathology in order to obtain reimbursement from third parties? How much of diagnosing is reality, and how much of it is conjecture arising from an outside authority who has decided what is and what is not a mental disorder? As Bacon (2018) insightfully states,

> Are there really 20 categories of mental illness, or 60, or 300, or 600? The only correct answer is that there are as many as the DSM committee believes there are and that number is not based on any independently verifiable foundation. In medicine, an X-ray confirms a broken bone and a blood test confirms diabetes; but there are no such real world correlates with mental health diagnoses. (p. 74)

Becoming aware of the therapy themes we create

When therapists understand that diagnosing, and psychotherapy itself, are constructed themes, they should heave a collective sigh of relief. If psychotherapy is a constructed theme not grounded in any distinct fundamental reality, then the therapist is left to create the session based on the interaction with the client. Now that we realize that therapy is just the construction of themes, we can focus on higher-level strength-based, resource-directed themes to move clients toward healing. By understanding that any interaction with clients is the creation or maintenance of a theme, therapists have the freedom to make new distinctions and to cocreate new themes with the clients rather than trying to fit clients into established themes.

For some therapists, the idea that therapy is a created in the moment may cause anxiety. So much of education about therapy is based on adhering to a specific method which does not deviate from the scripted theoretical interpretations. It is not uncommon to hear graduate-school professors encouraging their students to find a theory and to stick to it. The notion that the best intervention for a client is a moment-by-moment interaction is completely foreign to those who believe in a preplanned technique whatever the situation or whoever the client is. Evidence that shows that no specific theory works better than another and it is the interaction between client and therapist which creates change can make therapists feel as if they are drifting in a boat without a rudder and with no land in sight.

Creating new themes for clients requires therapists to be incredibly innovative and flexible. Preset actions and interpretations go by the wayside. To generate new themes that focus on client resources requires the therapist to shift from pathology to clients' strengths and potential. It involves moving clients out of their restricted themes and into expanded themes while paying less attention to the "problems." Once new themes are explored and accepted by clients, they will have access to the resourceful healing that resides inside themselves.

Psychotherapists generally use themes which react to clients' created themes. Most therapy themes are devised to combat the clients' initial distinctions. If clients say they have depression, therapists generally accept that theme. They then use other themes (theories) to eliminate the depression without recognizing they are working within the clients' theme of depression. No matter what technique or style the therapist uses, if it accepts and focuses on the client's theme, then therapy is stuck in a dichotomous pathology elimination. Simply relabeling symptoms into psycho-jargon does little to move attention away from what is perceived as the problem. It does not matter if the symptom is labeled defense mechanism, reactive attachment, cognitive distortion, or conditions of worth; if the interventions employed by therapists operate within the same theme, more attention is placed on the problem than on the potential strengths and resources clients may possess.

In spite of what many of us in the therapy profession might wish to believe, the therapist does not create change in clients. Therapists are not solely responsible for psychological adjustments in their clients, they are merely there to support and assist clients as clients change themselves. It is the client who finds the resources to create change. The therapists' role is to create the conditions for change to occur. Therapists are never completely responsible for the change that takes place in the client. Therapy is not a one-sided affair, but rather it has two sides, a cocreative process.

Bohart and Tallman (1999) presented the hypothesis that psychotherapy only really works because of the client. They state, "Clients are not submissive recipients of an intervention. They actively operate on therapists' inputs, transforming bits and pieces of the process into information and experiences which, in turn, are used to make change occur" (p. 95). It is the dynamic interaction between clients and therapists which produces a change in the levels of emotional arousal and helps clients to access their own inner resources for healing. Therapy is effective because clients utilize what has been offered to them in the interaction between themselves and the therapist. They then heal themselves. However, extensive interaction within themes of pathology and limitation are not empowering and only make it harder for clients to find those inner resources.

One individual who understood the importance of creating individualized resource-directed themes for his clients was the renowned psychiatrist, Milton Erickson. Erickson's method of creating change in his clients was considered not only innovative but radical. When he began practicing, the dominant view and practice of psychotherapy was based on the assumption that psychotherapy was a long and in-depth process. Clients were directed what to discuss by the therapists whose theoretical orientation placed priority on the interpretation of their clients' actions. The goal of therapy was to gain insight into the clients' problem's etiology because insight was what would create change. Through complicated procedures that delved into the clients' unconscious defense mechanisms, psychotherapists probed the clients' psyche to discover the hidden, unconscious motives for their emotions and behaviors. Advocates for this method believed that clients would change their behaviors once they knew what made them do what they did.

Erickson's approach was in complete opposition to the prevailing past-oriented views of therapy, and he believed in a more commonsense approach toward creating change. Erickson did not share the assumption that interpretation and insight would lead to change. Instead he believed that it was the therapy experience which clients had that led to change rather than the information they received. Erickson believed that the extensive investigation of clients' problems did little to alter those problems because constant attention on the problems often limited the clients' natural problem solving abilities (Haley, 1993; Leslie, 2014; O'Hanlon, 1987).

Also important was Erickson's respect for the individuality of each of his clients. Erickson saw each client as a unique individual, and he did not feel the need to have his clients conform to any predetermined model of therapy. He believed that each client needed to change in the way that was best for him or her, and should not be forced into any fixed prearranged techniques.

Erickson also avoided focusing on the clients' dysfunction and instead he focused on any potential strengths and resources that his clients possessed. He believed that it was the therapist's role to help clients find and use their own natural resources for growth and change. Erickson believed that clients often overlooked these resources and needed to be reminded of them as an aid in adapting to life's challenges. In essence, Erickson's method was a strategic process of helping his clients to design and accomplish their own personal goals (Short et al., 2005).

There is a good example of Erickson's unorthodox work with individuals and of how themes can be shifted. It is an often-cited case of his interaction with a disabled aunt of one of his colleagues who learned that Erickson was traveling to Milwaukee to give a lecture. This colleague had an aunt in Milwaukee who had experienced a series of health issues resulting in her being confined to a wheelchair. She lived alone in her mansion, had very little contact with the outside world, and had ceased all of her previous social activities including her regular and dedicated attendance at her church. Because of her isolation and her disability, the aunt was experiencing some form of depression. Her nephew was very worried about her and asked Erickson if he would check on her when he was in Milwaukee. Erickson agreed that, after his lecture, he would go visit his colleague's aunt.

When Erickson arrived at the aunt's home, he was warmly welcomed. The aunt gave him a tour of her large and elegant home. Erickson noticed that, other than adjustments which allowed the aunt to move around in her wheelchair, nothing had changed in the home for many years. The house was dark and it felt confining and depressing. He also mentally noted the pile of old church bulletins that were located in a corner of the living room. When she shared with Erickson her greenhouse nursery at the end of the house tour, the aunt perked up and glowed.

This nursery was a vibrant, colorful place where she spent hours working with many different plants. Erickson noticed that the walls of the greenhouse were lined with African violets. The aunt would take cuttings from these violets and then create other separate potted plants. Erickson, who had grown up on a farm, complimented her on her work and commented on how difficult it was to grow African violet plants from cuttings. The aunt appeared to appreciate Erickson's interest and his comments about her nursery, and Erickson quickly understood that the nursery was the only place where she felt a sense of contentment.

Erickson then disclosed that his real reason for the visit was because her nephew was very worried about her. She accepted his comments and agreed that she was indeed feeling very depressed. Surprisingly Erickson told her that he did not believe depression was her problem. Her problem was the fact that she had ceased performing her "Christian" duties. The aunt was very shocked by this comment and took offense. Erickson explained by telling her that she lived alone with a great deal of time and money available to her, and also had all of her beautiful plants. He said that she was wasting all of those wonderful gifts by simply staying alone in her home. Erickson then directed her to obtain the weekly bulletin from her church and to begin looking for all announcements regarding births, deaths, marriages, graduations, or anniversaries. She was to have her handyman drive her to visit the families mentioned in those announcements, and she should carry a potted clipping from her African violets to present as a gift.

After some thought, the aunt concurred with Erickson's assessment and promised to follow his instructions. After Erickson's visit, she began to visit people as Erickson had directed and, in time, she began to interact with people throughout her community. Many years later, when the aunt passed away, the local newspaper headline read, "African Violet Queen of Milwaukee Dies, Mourned by Thousands." For Erickson, rather than investigating her depression, it was more important to focus on and utilize the strengths and resources that the aunt had, her African violets and her faith (Gordon & Meyers-Anderson, 1981).

Erickson's work with the African Violet Queen is a wonderful example of how moving to a more resourceful theme can have a tremendous impact on clients. The depressed aunt was in the theme of "immobility, isolation, and depression." Erickson observed where she had energy and enthusiasm and merely shifted the theme of their interaction away from depression and toward "being a good Christian." This brilliant move changed the theme and the interaction within that theme. The aunt's desire to be a good Christian was much more empowering, resourceful, and effective than her previous theme of immobility, isolation, and depression. This one change in a theme transformed a lonely and solitary older woman into a renowned and inspiring figure in her city.

* * *

As we have seen, psychotherapy is a constructive endeavor. Traditional therapy is often based on the mental health practitioner's chosen theoretical approach rather than the uniqueness of the clients. These differing theories have all been shown to have successful outcomes, which lends little credibility to the idea that there is a "best" or "more effective" therapy. The majority of these theories are really problem-focused themes which have been constructed by theorists based on their own distinctions rather than any absolute fundamental reality. To generate healing, therapists must cocreate therapeutic themes with their clients which encourage clients' strengths and resources and activate their inner healing process. In the next chapter, we will discuss how therapists can shift the focus to resource-directed higher-order themes and away from lower-order techniques and applications.

CHAPTER 3

Cocreating new themes

In the previous chapter, we discussed how psychotherapy itself is often a constructed venture based on the therapists' preferred theories and techniques with little consideration of clients' unique and individual qualities. Since most styles of psychotherapy operate within problem-oriented themes, therapists often become trapped inside these limited themes. Therapists try to bring change for clients by repeating their own preferred theme (theory) instead of creating new empowering themes with their clients. However, it is the cocreation of new themes that center on the clients' strengths and resources which will help clients stimulate their own inner healing processes.

For the cocreation of new themes to occur, therapists must be comfortable directly relating to their clients rather than remaining as detached observers. Building new themes requires embracing a dynamic and interactive performance of therapy rather than by remaining faithful to any specific technical applications. Therapists must recognize that they are not the purveyors of ultimate truths about their clients. They will need to avoid the role of a separate observer who is uninvolved in therapeutic interaction. In a theme-creation view, psychotherapy is a relational process. Clients are the focus, with regard for their individual context. The recognition of clients' existing aptitudes and knowledge is crucial in designing new thematic interventions. These new themes can have immediate and surprising effects. As Papp and Imber-Black (1996) state, "Since themes address multiple levels of experience, it should come as no surprise that altering a central theme generates a process of change with widening effects in a fairly short period of time" (p. 19). In order to create new themes, the active participation by all parties is necessary. The primary concepts which aid in opening the space for new empowering themes to emerge are an emphasis on client resources, improvisation, and utilization.

Emphasizing resources

When constructing new themes in therapy, it is helpful to focus on themes which invite new possibilities. The easiest way to accomplish this is to first examine and then emphasize the resources that each client already possesses. A resource can be any set of client ideas, emotions, or actions that can be used to help activate their own inner healing. As Ray and Keeney (1993) state, "[A] resource is existentially meant any experience, belief, understanding, attitude, event, conduct, or interpersonal habit that contributes to the positive contextualization and realization of one's being" (p. 1).

By shifting the emphasis in therapy to client resources, it is easier to exit the client's disempowering themes. A resourceful theme opens up a new context for client behaviors and emotions that, at first, may appear to lack meaning or any positive connotations. A new theme is a new context in which established actions can generate new meanings. It is in the creation of a new theme that is guided by client resources that the door opens to the activation of client healing.

To access these resources, therapists must look for what clients have previously experienced that can be used to create new themes. This requires that therapists view the problematic themes brought to therapy as having the potential to become a resourceful theme. When therapy directs clients away from problem-oriented themes and toward their own inner resources, therapeutic interactions change from prearranged technique-driven discourses into spontaneous collaborations. Therapy can then move in surprising directions.

From this perspective, clients' problems are viewed as simply the loss of access to their own talents and virtues. In order to create new themes that reorient clients toward their resources, therapists must start wherever their clients are and then direct the discussion so that new empowering contexts and themes open up. If they listen intensely to the clients' descriptions, therapists will discover (1) the distinctions being created by clients and (2) potential escapes out of those limited descriptions. Since clients' themes are entrenched information systems, access to these systems must be through the introduction of stimulating but nonthreatening themes. Clients rarely protest when the discussion is about areas of their lives or actions which connect them to inspiring and energizing resources.

One of the main obstructions to moving out of problem-oriented themes is the therapist's own traditional unwavering focus on the client's problem. When both client and therapist are focused on what is problematic, creation of possibilities is limited. In addition, the use of regimented, standardized methods only makes matters worse since these are primarily problem-focused interventions. To help clients move toward their own inner healing, it is crucial that therapists move away from the prevailing problem-directed approaches that they have been taught. It requires a shift in the attention of both clients and therapists away from the problem to whatever can contribute positively to the clients' lives. From medicalized, pathology-based therapy, this appears to be counterintuitive because most psychotherapy training centers on the investigation of problems, the diagnosing of problems, and the predetermined therapy applications for those problems.

The more that information is elicited within a problem-oriented theme, often the harder therapists may find it to discover their clients' resources. When anything that could be used to exit from a limited theme presents itself, it is crucial that this potential resource be explored. As soon as a resource is detected, the client must be connected with that resource. This will facilitate a shift in the focus of the therapy session to a new theme which is connected to that resource.

Essentially, this approach to therapy emphasizes less stagnant problem exploration and more efforts to move clients out of problem-oriented themes so that clients can access resources and move beyond their problems. This requires that therapists guide sessions toward any resourceful themes which may appear. This will help clients to transfer their attention away from their problem-focused perspectives. By moving away from discussions of limitations while moving toward strengths and resources, therapists will have more freedom to explore other areas of their clients' lives. This shift could produce significant material to bring about positive therapeutic outcomes. When psychotherapy is focused only on pathology or dysfunction, the presence of beneficial, empowering client resources often goes unnoticed.

Anything clients bring to therapy has the potential to be a resource. An example of this is a session that I had with Taylor, a twenty-four-year-old male, who came to therapy for help with his overwhelming social anxiety. Taylor also brought his mother with him to my office. Even though he smiled and was friendly during our introductions, I could tell that he was a little anxious. As we began our session, Taylor told me that he had been diagnosed with autism when he was eighteen years old and had been told that he had Asperger's syndrome. He told me that he had brought his mother with him because of his anxiety when meeting new people. He felt that his mother was a calming influence when he entered new situations. Taylor described the history of his trials and tribulations with anxiety. He said that he became overwhelmed with worry very quickly when he met and interacted with new people. Taylor said that he even sometimes felt anxious when interacting with people that he already knew. He admitted to being relieved when he was diagnosed with autism because this was a legitimate reason for his behavior. Now he didn't feel that he was "really crazy," which had previously concerned him.

Even though Taylor had an explanation for the cause of his anxiety, he still desperately wanted to be less anxious around other people. He told me that he presently lived with his mother and father who were understanding of his condition. At home he felt safe and did not have much anxiety, but he would often become very anxious around others in a variety of other settings. This anxiety had caused him much stress during his early years in school. Taylor had also found that his social anxiety was problematic for him when working at a job because he had to interact with the other employees. He really wanted to be comfortable around people, but he felt that an alarm would go off in his mind if he got too close to others and this caused overwhelming fear. Taylor's gaze drifted away from me as he looked out the window. "It can be terrifying for me to have to be around people I don't know well. Once I get to know them, I am still a little anxious, but I can handle it better." The initial theme of the first session clearly was "People Are Terrifying" with Taylor playing the starring role.

Taylor's mother said that growing up, he frequently had to stay out of school for extended periods of time due to his anxiety. However, according to her, in spite of his fear, it appeared that people liked Taylor and that most people were understanding of his condition. He often assisted with running the soundboard for the music program at their church on Sundays, and he had always done a good job. Other than playing video games at home alone, it appeared that running the soundboard was one of the few activities that Taylor seemed to really enjoy and to have less anxiety about. Both Taylor and his mother felt stuck in this situation and were unable to move past the autism-related anxiety which Taylor had experienced for most of his life.

Hearing about the soundboard at church, I immediately seized on it as a potential resource for Taylor. "Do you like music?" I asked him. He replied that he did. "Do you play any musical instruments?" I asked him. Taylor shyly smiled and said, "I am trying to learn to play the bass guitar." "Are you taking lessons?" I asked. "No. I just try to figure it out on my own." I told Taylor that I was impressed that he had such a good ear for music and inquired what songs he had been learning. Taylor's shyness slowly began to disappear as he told me that he recently was learning how to play the famous rock and roll song "Smoke on the Water" by the band Deep Purple. "Really?" I exclaimed. "That sounds pretty amazing. In time, I am sure you will learn quite a few other songs." Our discussion continued into the realm of music as Taylor told me about the type of bass guitar that he owned and what other brands he would like to own one day. He seemed to relax more as he talked about the differing types of amplifiers and how he could run them through the soundboard at his church. He also talked about the different songs he would like to learn and the variety of genres of music that he also enjoyed.

I could see that music was a positive resource in Taylor's life, but also saw that he was not fully immersing himself in it. It was important to get Taylor to occupy his mind with something other than his anxiety about people, and music appeared to be the best option. When Taylor paused from his comments about music, I asked him, "Have you thought about playing in a band?" Taylor's face showed a mixture of curiosity and interest. "I never thought about playing in a band," he said. I could now see that there was a small spark of interest. "Taylor, it might be fun being a bass player in a band. Bass players sit back and groove to the music. They don't stand up in front of everyone like a singer or a guitar player." I was hoping that Taylor would continue to be curious about my comments as I opened up a new theme which involved something Taylor liked to do, play music. I also honored the presence of his anxiety in the idea of playing in a band noting that he could stay in the background. Taylor seemed intrigued by my comment. "I guess that would be fun if I didn't have to be in front of everyone." At that point, I knew I had a resource to help move Taylor out of his theme of "People Are Terrifying."

"Taylor, the more I think about this problem, the more I think that this is not a problem of your being afraid as much as it is a problem of not having an outlet for your creativity," I told him with a very serious look. "I understand that some of your anxiety may be due to the autism, but I really think that some of your anxiety may be tied to your not having a place to put all your creative energy. Some people have excess amounts of creative energy, and when they don't have anything to do with it, this energy piles up, and it can feel like anxiety. I wonder if you had a place to focus your extra creative energy, then perhaps you might see a decrease in anxiety."

I then talked to Taylor and his mother about how anxiety is often mislabeled and confused with nervous excitement. I did not negate what Taylor was feeling. I provided an alternative explanation for his anxious feeling and suggested that perhaps those feelings were not all bad. I asked Taylor if he would be happy if his anxiety were to decrease even by only about twenty percent. He told me that he would be happy with any decrease. I told Taylor and his mother that my clinical intuition was telling me that playing music was an effective way to decrease some of his anxiety and instead put it to a positive and enjoyable use. The theme of therapy began to shift away from "People Are Terrifying" toward a new theme of "Channeling Creative Energy into Music."

I then wondered out loud if perhaps Taylor would progress faster with his bass guitar playing if he took music lessons. His mother said that the director of the music programs at their church also gave lessons. I turned to Taylor and asked if he liked the music director. Taylor said yes, he liked the music director and thought that they worked well together. Things began falling into place once we began to move out of the anxiety-based theme. I asked Taylor if he would be interested in taking two lessons with the music director. I specifically asked for "two lessons" because it was a lower, less anxiety-provoking number for Taylor rather than a long-term commitment to taking lessons. For almost a full minute Taylor sat quietly thinking. He then looked at me and said, "I don't think it would hurt to take a lesson or two." I told him that, with his natural talent, he should progress fairly quickly. I even joked that he was training for a future career as a rock-and-roll star who sits in the background. Our therapeutic goal for the next week was for Taylor to contact the church music director to inquire about taking lessons. Taylor's mother pledged to pay for the first two lessons and agreed that it would be a good outlet for Taylor's nervous energy. Taylor seemed a little hesitant, but he still appeared intrigued by the idea of playing more music to decrease his anxiety.

Two weeks later I was told by Taylor's mother that he had taken two lessons, and he really liked learning from the music director. She told me that even though he was very nervous about interacting one-on-one with his new music teacher, he discovered that they got along very well. His teacher even told Taylor that if he continued to progress, the director might someday want him to play with the church music group during the services. Taylor's mother was surprised that Taylor had hinted that he might be open to playing with the church group. Taylor said that if he did play with the group, the director told him that he could stay in the background.

Within a month of first coming to therapy, Taylor reported his anxiety levels slowly decreasing as he interacted more often with his music teacher. He also found that, even though he would still get very nervous, he slowly became more open to talking with other people at the church. He diligently practiced his bass guitar and put more of his energy into learning his music. This also appeared to help him focus his mind a little more. In time, Taylor began to question some of his automatic fears about interacting with others after his experiences of playing music and became even more involved in his church. The last time I heard from

Taylor's mother she told me that, even though he still experiences higher levels of anxiety due to his autism, he did not feel as if he were in a daily battle with his fear. She also told me he was getting quite good at the bass guitar and becoming more open to playing in his church. The use of the resource of music led to a new theme which opened the door for Taylor to have interactions with others and to learn to deal with his anxiety more effectively. It is possible that, due to his autism, Taylor may always have a higher-level of anxiety, but operating out of a more resourceful theme gave him some tools to focus his energy and to make new connections.

Improvisation

In order to quickly shift attention toward new themes, it is important that therapists are open to improvisation. Creating new themes requires a therapeutic performance that is free from any preparation or predetermined therapeutic interventions. Interaction between therapist and client is an alive, present-moment engagement so therapists' actions should be unrehearsed and spontaneous. Anything offered by that interaction which can help move clients out of their limiting themes must be employed in the moment. To accomplish this, therapists must first learn to let go of any rigid ideas of how therapy is to proceed. By incorporating improvisation, sessions can become much more spirited and inspired.

Spontaneously created themes are the offering of new distinctions based on information obtained from the client. When introducing new distinctions, it is important that therapists observe their clients' immediate feedback to determine if the new theme has resonated. Since there are a plethora of distinctions that can be drawn about any one event, the therapist should not be locked into any one specific theme. If one distinction does not resonate with the client, the therapist then moves on to the next opportunity to open up the session to new ideas and perspectives. By not being confined into any specific theoretical orientation, therapists have the freedom to flow with the present moment. Since themes are constructed in the immediate interaction between client and therapist, this allows, and requires, a unique method to be used for each client. As Papp and Imber-Black (1996) point out, because themes are "embedded in a different form of logic, they are capable of releasing the therapist from conventional and redundant ways of thinking" (p. 17).

Famed acting coach, Viola Spolin (1999), viewed improvisation as a way to resolve problems without any predetermination of how it will be done while allowing anything in the environment to aid in the resolution. Openness to the present moment without clinging to fixed ideas can create space for new ideas. In allowing anything into the therapeutic interaction, possibilities will present themselves which can lead to new resource-rich themes that will benefit clients.

To create a major shift in clients' patterns, therapists must be at ease with improvisational actions that are often unexpected and can appear random to their clients. The same old information stated in the same old way usually has the same old effect. However, when clients allow unique and out-of-the-ordinary information into their perceived reality, then their reality has to rearrange itself and accommodate the new information. This introduction of something random can cause a shift in how clients relate to and respond to their problems.

The presentation of random information can come from almost anywhere; however, it rarely ever comes from preplanned procedures. When therapists relax and allow room for spontaneity, openings can appear and therapeutic themes can transform. Constant problem investigation will not elicit new information because excessive examination of problems only provides therapists and clients with old information. The way out of disempowering themes is to permit the introduction of new material within a lively interaction. This will facilitate movement away from old themes based on any perceived limitations and disempowerment.

Therapists will find that some of their spontaneous interventions may at first appear strange or absurd to their clients. Random information can initially create a feeling of confusion in clients because it is unexpected. However, the unexpected creates shifts in the clients' narratives and interrupts their habitual ways of thinking and feeling. New possibilities emerge. Something strange and random can also bypass the clients' excessively analytic thinking which might dismiss attempts at solving their problems.

Therapeutic improvisation not only opens a space for new ideas, it also permits both clients and therapists to authentically connect.

Trust between the two parties is fostered. When spontaneous actions and perceptions are fostered and appreciated, clients are encouraged to let go of their attempts at control. Improvisation in therapy also can help clients to enlarge their perspectives of what is possible as they move away from their own previous problem-oriented evaluations (Farley, 2017; Galvez & Crouch, 2017). When improvisation is permitted into the therapeutic interaction, a cocreative process between clients and therapists can emerge which transcends problems.

The potential for this cocreative process is sometimes limited when therapists attempt to force specific techniques or actions into a session. Allowing the session to "go with the flow" gives rise to new possibilities and outcomes. Many therapists may be uncomfortable with the real possibility of their therapy sessions moving into unknown areas. However, it is in these unknown areas where new possibilities for transforming themes may hide. By welcoming in the unknown, therapists increase their options for utilizing new information which may help create new themes.

Here is an example of being open to anything which presents itself in a session. I had a session with Grant, a thirty-two-year-old father, and his twelve-year-old son, Wyatt. Grant had come to see me twice before to discuss the trouble he was having in connecting with Wyatt. Grant had been absent for most of Wyatt's childhood due to his own struggles, with addiction. He had finally been able to break free from his demons and for the past two years had been diligently trying to be a good father to Wyatt. Wyatt's mother had forgiven Grant for his past actions, and they had united on co-parenting as best they could. The problem was that Wyatt was understandably distant and resentful toward Grant because of Grant's absence and his inconsistent parenting over the years. Wyatt talked very little about his feelings, and Grant felt that he was often stonewalled when he tried to talk to Wyatt about their relationship.

Grant brought Wyatt to session in the hopes that we could create some sort of dialogue between the three of us about Wyatt's feelings toward Grant. Even though Wyatt appeared initially very friendly when we were introduced, by the time we settled into my office Wyatt had erected a wall which seemed impenetrable. He gave one-word answers to questions. He was very resistant to making much eye contact when we began discussing what Grant had hoped for the session to produce. I could see why it was difficult to connect with Wyatt. He was fully committed to not talking about what made him feel uncomfortable or resentful. Within five minutes the session had come to a screeching halt.

Grant was frustrated at Wyatt's lack of involvement, and I could sympathize; however, I felt that pushing Wyatt would not help Wyatt's mood. It was also ineffective in opening communication. I immediately redirected Grant and Wyatt to small talk. I told them I just wanted to get to know both of them a little bit before we started diving into therapeutic work. Both seemed a little relieved to move away from the seriousness of the reason for their arrival in there.

I was at a loss for how to approach the situation so I began to ask both of them what they enjoyed doing in their free time. Grant told me he enjoyed fishing because it was relaxing to him. Wyatt told me that he had been playing video games for similar reasons. I then inquired if they had any hobbies together. Both denied having any mutual hobbies, but something told me to persist in my questioning about activities that they enjoyed. They both thought for a moment and shook their heads. Suddenly Wyatt smiled and said, "We both like to watch wrestling!" My clinical intuition told me to grab hold of this nugget of information and improvise.

I determined that Wyatt was referring to "professional wrestling" which is a televised choreographed performance in which athletes supposedly compete in violent wrestling matches which involve acrobatics and scripted dialogues. This form of wrestling is solely entertainment and has little resemblance to Olympic-style wrestling. Many of the professional wrestlers portray flamboyant and eccentric characters who engage in over-the-top theatrics while exhibiting athletic prowess. I remembered watching wrestling when I was young boy.

I seized on this information and began to ask Wyatt what he liked about watching wrestling. Wyatt began to open up as he talked about his favorite wrestlers and the recent storylines that were taking place on the programs he watched. I noticed that Grant was starting to smile. He watched his son as Wyatt became a bit excited as he talked about how much he enjoyed watching wrestling. I asked Wyatt if he thought Grant liked watching it as well. Wyatt quickly said that he did and named the wrestlers that Grant preferred along with their backgrounds. I was surprised at how much Wyatt had come alive once we began talking about wrestling. I also noticed that he was making more eye contact with me and with his father. I felt that I needed to utilize this newly found resource that the father and son shared.

I turned to Grant and asked him if he agreed with Wyatt's assessment of his favorite wrestlers. Grant lit up with a bigger smile and concurred with Wyatt's comments. I asked him what he thought of being able to watch wrestling with his son. He stated that he really enjoyed the two of them being able to sit down and just relax while watching these programs. Grant felt that it was probably the only thing they really got to enjoy together. Wyatt chimed in saying that he and Grant also teased each other about the other's favorite wrestler and would sometimes bet each other about which wrestler would win. At that point, an idea popped into my mind that seemed a little silly at first, but proved to be a turning point, not just in the session, but in Grant and Wyatt's relationship.

"You know what just occurred to me?" I asked Grant and Wyatt. They both shook their heads. "I think you two are like a tag team in wrestling!" I was referring to a wrestling performance in which two wrestlers form a team and face off against another two-man team. "It is like you two are so into this stuff that you could be a tag team yourselves." Grant and Wyatt laughed. "I really mean it" I told them. "It is as if you both know the right thing to say and do when you are watching and analyzing this stuff." Grant laughed again and said, "Yeah, we really enjoy it. Good mindless entertainment." Wyatt nodded his head in agreement with his father's comment.

"Wyatt, do you think you could talk like one of those wrestlers when they start talking to the television camera?" I asked. Wyatt became still and seemed to not understand what I was asking him. "Do you remember when those wrestlers have a microphone and talk about an upcoming match? You remember when they are ranting and threatening to beat up whoever is in the next match? Do you think you could do that?" Wyatt then smiled and told me he probably could. I then asked him if he could do it as his favorite wrestler. Wyatt then laughed, but was hesitant. I told him that I would go first. I stood up and put on a totally ridiculous performance as a loud fictitious wrestler telling his fans that he was going to easily beat up all his challengers because of a combination of strength and good looks. I grabbed an unopened bottle of water and used it as a mock microphone. My childhood memories of watching wrestling came in handy as I gave an intentionally over-the-top spontaneous performance.

Both Grant and Wyatt's eyes widened, and they laughed as I finished. "Do you think you could do that Wyatt?" I asked, hoping that my performance had given my clients permission to act a little silly. Wyatt agreed to act as his favorite wrestler. As he stood up, I handed him the water bottle to use as his microphone. He launched into a very funny and accurate impression of a wrestler. I marveled at how Wyatt had suddenly come alive and seemed to really be good at the impromptu performance. I then turned to Grant and said, "Since Wyatt and I have given our wrestlers a voice, how about you?" Grant smiled, but looked unsure. I silently nodded my head to nonverbally encourage him. He agreed and the water bottle microphone was passed to him.

Initially, Grant did not display the energy of my or Wyatt's performance and he seemed a little uncomfortable acting so silly. However, he came alive when suddenly Wyatt shouted out, "Come on, Dad!" Grant began to get into the fun and yelled silly things into the water bottle microphone. He stomped around and threatened other wrestlers and touted his own incredible wrestling abilities. When he had finished his performance, both Wyatt and I applauded. "Wow! I did not know you had that in you!" I told him. Both father and son laughed and smiled at each other. This was certainly not something that they (or I) had expected to happen in their session.

"I really want you two to play a wrestling tag team now," I said. "I would like to hear you guys do this as if you have an upcoming match against some other tag team … let's call them the Destroyers." Grant and Wyatt looked at me slightly puzzled until Wyatt suddenly seized the opportunity and starting talking to his father with his wrestling persona. "Listen up!" he said loudly. "We are going to take on the Destroyers and destroy them! I am going to do my part and win this match!" Wyatt's quick entrance into his wrestling persona surprised Grant and me, but we encouraged him to go on. Wyatt then talked about specific wrestling moves this fictitious tag team would use and how it would help them win.

When Wyatt finished his commentary, Grant started in with his wrestling persona. Grant was as lively as Wyatt, and I found myself amazed at how quickly he picked up where Wyatt had left off. Grant got into his performance and matched what Wyatt had done. He was even more animated in his performance than previously. Father and son were interacting as a real tag team.

Grant finished his wrestling soliloquy. Wyatt immediately jumped back in and started telling Grant that he would have to have the right moves or they would lose their fight. I noticed that now both Grant and Wyatt seemed to have forgotten that I was in the room as they went back and forth with their wrestling banter. I also noticed that some of the things Wyatt was beginning to say could be related to the relationship issues that he and his father had. Wyatt began to tell Grant that he wasn't sure he could depend on Grant because the opponents they would face were very tough. This may have been standard wrestling dialogue, but it seemed to come from a place close to Wyatt's heart.

Grant responded to Wyatt's questioning of his dependability. Grant told him that he would be right there with Wyatt in the match and he would do anything he could to win it. Wyatt became a little more forceful in his reply. "I can't trust you because you didn't have my back in the last match! I had to fight them all by myself. I didn't know where you were!" exclaimed Wyatt. I was hearing Wyatt's hurt come out but safely masked in a silly role play about professional wrestling. I think Grant heard it as well because he hesitated for a moment before replying. "Listen! I know I was not good at having your back when we were in that match, but I swear this time is different. I got your back! I will be there to defeat the Destroyers. They can't beat us if we stay together!" said Grant passionately.

Wyatt suspiciously looked at Grant and continued to put on his show as a wrestler by questioning if Grant had the strength and courage to fight alongside him. Even though both parties were still in their fictional personas, it appeared that both were starting to say to each other what they had always wanted to say. Grant paused for another moment. He then looked into Wyatt's eyes and told him, "Champ, if you will allow me another chance to get in the ring with you, I promise I will protect you when you are tagged into the match. I promise that I will make sure that you and I win that match. I know I have not been a good tag team partner in the past, but I got the right moves now and I know that I am up for the job." Wyatt became quiet and nodded his head.

Not wanting to lose the momentum, I playfully interjected to Wyatt, "I don't know about this guy. He seems to want to win, but how can you trust him?" "I don't know if I can," Wyatt replied in his wrestler voice. "He says this but when the match is on anything can happen." "That is true," I said. "Maybe you just have to test him out to see if he is up to the task of being your partner." Grant turned to me and earnestly said in his own voice, "I know I am up for it." Wyatt looked at me, and I nodded to him. "Maybe we should give this guy a shot?" Wyatt shrugged his shoulder with a slight smile. The performance was now over.

I told Grant and Wyatt that I thought that their performance was excellent and that I knew in my heart that they could be a successful tag team. We finished our session by talking about what specifically makes a successful tag team. I asked both Grant and Wyatt how they would know if they could be a successful team in dealing with life. Wyatt expressed a little more in the session than he had when he arrived, and Grant appeared to be more relaxed. Both contributed ideas about how to work together a little more effectively. When the session came to a close, I asked both of them to take notes the next time they watched a wrestling program and to bring them to the next session. I wanted them to write out what specifically the wrestlers were doing to be successful in their matches. Both agreed to follow the directive and left the session.

Two weeks later, Grant came to his next session without Wyatt since the boy had an after-school activity that he was required to complete. Once we sat down in my office, Grant broke into a huge grin. "You just won't believe what happened, Doc!" he stated. "Wyatt and I have been spending more time together and we are really getting along better. I don't know what happened in the last session, but since then he has been really more open to me and talks to me a little more. It is like he isn't so angry with me. I don't want to get my hopes up, but I have to tell you, things are really a lot better."

Grant also said that he and Wyatt had done the assignment of writing down what the successful wrestlers did to win their matches. Grant and Wyatt agreed that the wrestlers controlled their emotions, waited until the right time to make their finishing moves, and never gave up. He said that they still watched wrestling, but they also had started doing other things together. He and Wyatt had gone fishing together the previous week, and it had been fun for both of them. Grant seemed genuinely surprised at how much things had changed. He was aware that there was still plenty of work to do to gain more trust from Wyatt, but he reveled in the fact that Wyatt was interested in doing something with him other than simply watching wrestling.

In time, Grant and Wyatt became closer and found that they could depend on each other a little more. The improvisation of talking like wrestlers appeared to give both parties a safe way to express what they felt while opening the door to a new theme for them. I truly feel that the seeds of reconciliation were planted in their playful wrestling interaction, and this would not have happened for Grant and Wyatt if there had not been an openness in the session for something out of the ordinary. It was by improvising on a resourceful connection between the two that the session was enabled to move out of the theme of "The Son Who Will Not Forgive" and into the new theme of "The Successful Tag Team."

Utilization

Utilization is necessary for the transformation of themes and requires that therapists view anything brought forth by their clients as tools that can be used to create therapeutic change. From this perspective, therapists are encouraged to take any client action or experience and use it to move the focus of the therapy session away from distressed themes. Instead of struggling with the clients' patterns of emotion and behavior, utilization becomes a creative process for incorporating those patterns into an improvised approach for change. Anything that happens in the interaction between therapist and client can be used to move toward resource-oriented themes of interaction, whether it is resistance, frustration, or reaction. No matter what happens therapists can employ it for therapeutic change.

Therapists who practice utilization must be open to the possibility that whatever they are given can become a helpful resource to facilitate transformation. When therapists adjust their approach to embrace what is happening at that moment, rather than struggle against what is unexpected and may be undesirable, openings toward client resources can magically appear. Forcing clients into the therapists' own worldview does little more than limit the possibilities for change and also harms the therapeutic relationship. A key to using what clients bring to create more inspiring themes is first of all the initial validation of the clients' experiences. Clients are much more open to changing direction when they feel it is not being forced on them.

In order to incorporate what a client offers us in the interaction, we have to be creative and open. By looking for positive intentions on the part of clients, therapists can more easily change the limiting distinctions which the clients have assigned to themselves. This can then lead to an easier exit out of the clients' restrictive themes. For example, a client who has a very cautious nature could be redesignated instead as someone who takes his time to thoroughly understand a situation before making a decision. A client who always has to be right could be described as someone who has the courage to fight for her own personal truth. A client who is often emotional may be a person who is courageous enough to allow himself to feel his emotions. A client who compulsively checks the locks on her door multiple times a day could even be praised for caring about the safety of her family. All of these examples are possibilities for entering into new themes which use what is already present in the clients to work toward obtaining positive outcomes. Rather than fighting against a symptom, the therapist will employ what is provided by the client to creatively find new ways to assist the client in healing.

The therapeutic use of utilization is found in the work of Milton Erickson. One of Erickson's more well-known examples of the use of utilization was his work with a male patient at the hospital where Erickson once worked. The patient claimed to be Jesus Christ and was not swayed by any attempts to convince him otherwise. Erickson approached him one day and told him that since the man was Jesus Christ, he understood that he had experience working as a carpenter. The man immediately agreed with Erickson's comment. Erickson then asked the man if it was true that the man had come to be of service to people. The man immediately told Erickson he had. Erickson then asked the man if he could assist in the building of some new furniture that was needed at the hospital. The man agreed and began helping construct some bookshelves for the hospital. This change of pattern of behavior in the man led to better interactions with other patients and hospital staff and a decrease in the severity of his symptoms. Rather than fight against the man's problem, Erickson chose to use it as a way to facilitate change.

Utilization can also involve things that are not directly related to the client but which present themselves during the session. Being open to whatever occurs helps to welcome in opportunities to use random information to exit limited themes. I once had a bird perch outside my office and began to sing loudly. When I asked my client what he thought about the bird singing, he replied that "Birds must enjoy life because they are always singing." This led to a discussion about how he could begin metaphorically singing through his own life. Another time a comment from a client about a bright color in the room led to a conversation about how she could add more "sparkle" to her life. Utilizing what shows up in the therapy session requires therapists to be open to the random and be willing to leave behind predetermined plans for how the therapeutic discourse should unfold.

I once worked with a woman whom I will call Juanita. She came to therapy because of her despair over the strained relationship she had with two of her adult children. Juanita had tried desperately to please all of her children while they were growing up. However, due to her constant caretaking and enabling, they had grown into entitled and self-centered adults who cared little about their mother's feelings. Juanita freely admitted that her adult children's present behavior was her fault. She gave them whatever they wanted so that they would never suffer or want for anything. She had done most of this as a single mother after her husband's death when the children were little. It became obvious to me that Juanita was a hardworking, motivated person who seemed to care about the welfare of everyone in her life, but she had little desire or energy to devote to herself.

In our discussions, I noticed that any attempt on my part to point out where Juanita could be practicing self-care using some of the energy she had used to please her children was usually disregarded or ignored. She had a long history of doing more than she should have done for those close to her. Unfortunately, she felt overwhelmed and disappointed when her well-meaning actions were not reciprocated. It appeared to me that no suggestions or directives would initiate a change in Juanita's pattern of always putting others before herself. It was almost as if her entire identity was centered on her selfless and martyred behavior. I have learned that once a person begins to identify with the problem, it can often be a tricky affair to get them to change because of their resistance. This is because any amount of change to their problem may result in resistance. This resistance is based on their unconscious belief that a change in the problem (which they identify with) indirectly means a change in who clients think they are. If there is any perception, conscious or unconscious, that people may lose their sense of identity, they naturally avoid change because the existential anxiety connected with a loss of identity can be overpowering. I felt this was the case with Juanita. She had been identifying herself as a person who was a selfless giver. She had acquiesced for so long that even a small adjustment from the outside quickly met with dismissal or avoidance.

I decided that the best route to get her to value herself more was to utilize something that she often talked about in her session, her Catholic faith. Juanita had been raised in a deeply religious household and both of her parents had been very active members of the Catholic Church. Juanita continued practicing her Catholic faith as an adult and often told me how much her religion meant to her. She told me that every Saturday evening she would create a new shrine in her home that had pictures of the saints, candles, and incense. Every week she would also put a picture in her shrine of someone whom she believed needed help. She prayed for them daily over the course of that week. Juanita would make time every evening to sit in front of her shrine and say her daily prayers and perform other rituals related to her faith. She told me that she took time to think about the good qualities of the person who needed help and to think good thoughts about them. Outside of her children, her daily prayers were the most important part of her life.

I decided to utilize Juanita's daily prayers at her shrine to get her to at least consider that she had value as a person also. As she was again talking about her children and their present disagreements, I suddenly interrupted her with the comment, "I am really very worried about your children." Juanita stopped and looked surprised. She asked me why I had said that. I looked down at the floor with a very concerned look on my face and said, "I worry about them because I just don't know what they are going to do if something happens to you. I worry that you could become ill and not be able to continue to help them. I mean, God forbid, something worse could even happen. I see it all the time. I am not trying to frighten you, Juanita, but I just hope you stay healthy." Juanita was taken aback by my comments. She wanted to know why I had thought about her children that way. I explained that the future is not promised to any of us, and I have seen many good people unable to help their loved ones due to changes in their own lives. I knew that raising her children without her husband, Juanita was well aware of how difficult things could be for families when life takes unexpected turns.

Juanita sat quietly for a moment pondering what I had said. I then told Juanita how much I admired her dedication to her family and how much she cared for them. I told her that the world can be such an uncertain place, and we could only hope for the best for all the good people in the world. Juanita began agreeing with me when I praised her care for her children and asserted the undeniable fact that the future is uncertain for all. I then asked her how she deals with the uncertainty of life. As I expected, she told me that her faith helped her to cope with life's uncertainty, and it had been a tremendous source of strength for her during very tough times. I nodded in agreement to her comments and told her that not many people have such a strong faith as she. I also told her that it was possible that her praying for those in her shrine had helped many people over the years. She smiled and told me that she felt that her prayers were heard by God and that God helps those who believe in him.

I then asked Juanita if she would do me a favor. She nodded without hesitation. I asked her if she would be willing to put a picture of herself on her shrine for the next two weeks. Would she pray that she would continue to have good physical and mental health so that she could continue helping her children? She was a little taken aback by my request because she had always only put other people who needed help into her shrine. I told her that I completely understood, but if she were to pray to God about herself the same way she prayed for everyone else, it might help her stay healthy and safe so that she could help others more effectively. It took a little convincing on my part, but Juanita eventually agreed to my request and promised to place a small picture of herself on her shrine. I let her know that by connecting to God in the way that she had been doing, there was a chance that she could get spiritual assistance in maintaining her own health so that she could continue to help the important people in her life. I knew that the only way to get her to take time to think about herself in any positive manner was to utilize what she was already doing. The theme of therapy moved from "Problems with My Entitled Adult Children" to "Connecting with God to Better Help Others." Juanita left our session with a promise to place her photo on her shrine Saturday evening and pray for herself over the next two weeks the same way she had been praying for others who had needed help.

When Juanita returned to her next therapy session, she told me how she had diligently followed my request and had put her picture on her shrine for the past two weeks. She said that she had prayed daily to God for her to continue her good health. She also had thought about the good qualities she possessed and how she could be of service to others. She reported feeling a little more positive about herself in general. She admitted that praying for herself was something that she had rarely done in the past. After praying for herself for two weeks she noticed that she was feeling more focused about what was important to her. She told me that she had begun to realize that she was spending too much time worrying about her children when there were other people whom she could be helping and who might even need her more. Taking the time to pray for her health made her think more about taking better care of herself. She had begun to change some of the habits that were detrimental to her. She had stopped snacking on sugary foods in the evening and had spent more time walking around her neighborhood. Juanita also began checking on a neighbor who was having some health issues to see if she could be of assistance. She told me that her neighbor had been very appreciative and invited Juanita over for coffee one afternoon, and they both had enjoyed chatting with one another. They began talking frequently, and Juanita had started helping her neighbor by running errands that were difficult for the neighbor. Juanita found that she began looking forward to checking on her neighbor after she got off work. The neighbor seemed to genuinely appreciate Juanita's efforts to help.

The issues with her adult children still bothered Juanita, but she was not as distraught or angry with the situation as she had been two weeks earlier. It appeared that indirectly focusing on herself helped to redirect Juanita's energy away from the constant demands of her entitled children and more toward her primary goal in life, which was to help others. By utilizing her weekly shrine construction and daily prayers, I was able to get Juanita to do what she might otherwise have easily dismissed had I directed her to do this. In time, Juanita started checking in on several of her neighbors and focusing less on her children's demands.

* * *

Emphasizing resources, improvisation, and utilization are all necessary ingredients in transforming therapeutic themes. These concepts, when woven together, help free therapeutic discourse from the chains of pathology-focused interventions. By allowing new and surprising action into sessions, therapists will find that the therapy process can take remarkable turns which neither therapist nor client could expect. In permitting a flow of interaction that is spontaneous and unscripted, new distinctions can more easily be formed and new opportunities for growth can present themselves. The construction of new themes requires equal participation of clients and therapists as each reacts and responds to the other. It is in these lively interactions that new meanings surface, new contexts emerge, and healing commences. In the next chapter we will discuss pragmatic actions therapists can take to encourage the changing of themes in therapy.

CHAPTER 4

Thematic patterns and rituals

Previously we covered how resources, improvisation, and utilization are vital components of a theme-oriented approach to psychotherapy. By permitting more lively interaction and creativity to permeate therapy sessions, therapists are better able to use the clients' own resources to construct more energizing themes. These concepts shift clients away from pathology-focused themes and into more resource-oriented perspectives which help them find their own solutions. As discussed earlier, psychotherapy is too often focused on categorical descriptions of emotions and behavior. Therapists sometimes find themselves held fast in classification systems constructed of generalizations with labels based on rigid frames of reference. In a traditional "talk" therapy perspective, we are also frequently hindered by our own language. We think our words or phrases are concrete entities that create similar meanings for everyone who hears them. We forget that any meaning is created or discovered through how one interprets all incoming information. This interpretation then attaches us to a distinct perception of reality. Kirmayer (1993) reminds us that meaning is "not a thing or substance; it is a term for the active relationship of receiver to message or—since we are not only receivers of meaning but equally its creators—of self to world" (p. 162).

Since our language is structured by our social and cultural perspectives, it behooves therapists to find new ways to move past our language to seek methods of change. The unconscious mind operates in symbolic representations which are beyond our socially constructed language and may offer much more flexibility as we work toward change. When "conscious mind-oriented therapy" approaches have limited results, therapists should proceed to the hidden, symbolic domain of the unconscious mind to bring about change. Two effective concepts beyond strictly "conscious therapy" applications are (1) the use of pattern alterations and (2) therapeutic rituals. These concepts can create new experiences for clients that may increase their behavioral flexibility and open space for new transformational themes to arise.

Pattern alterations

Clients want to find solutions to their problems, but they are often unaware that their attempts to create a solution operate within the same theme in which they experience their problem. This can lead to feeling stuck when repeated attempts to solve the problem appear futile. Often the actions taken to solve their problem only continue to solidify its existence and strengthen the overall theme into which they are locked. As Rohrbaugh and Shoham (2001) point out,

> Whether occurring within or between people, these processes persist because problem and attempted solution become intertwined in a vicious cycle, or positive feedback loop, in which more of the solution leads to more of the problem, leading to more of the same solution, and so on. (p. 66)

As many of the early developers of brief therapy asserted, it is often the very methods that clients are using to change their problems that contribute the most to the preservation of those specific problems (Fisch et al., 1982; Hale & Frusha, 2016).

The clients' attempts to change their problematic patterns frequently end in disappointment. Since the patterns are performed with regularity, they have become unconscious processes that appear to happen automatically. These unconscious processes are very challenging to change through traditional talk therapy because they take place outside of the clients' conscious awareness. Clients do not always know when the process will occur or how to stop its activation. Any attempt to change these patterns often results in a paradox for clients because, (1) it is not possible to consciously know what is unconscious, and (2) any effort to change the pattern requires conscious thought of the pattern which could activate it.

Instead of directing clients toward ceasing the habitual behavior and potentially evoking resistance, it is often best to adjust just one small part of the habitual pattern. Even a small adjustment can lead to long-term changes. To start this adjustment, therapists must first view client problems not as frozen pathological states but as processes which clients unconsciously initiate. The alteration of any part of this process could change the clients' ability to experience the problem in their accustomed manner. This hampers their ability to continue in the same operating theme. The altering of the execution of their patterns can directly change their problematic theme.

Excessive time spent determining where and why the problem originated does not give detailed information on how specifically clients are experiencing their problems. While always honoring the clients' narratives, therapists must also know: (1) where the problem occurs, (2) when it usually happens, (3) how long it persists, (4) who is the client with when it occurs, and (5) any other important particulars that could be helpful. It is crucial that therapists obtain as much information as possible about their clients' experiences with their problems. Paying attention to clients' behavioral patterns is important since these patterns may be the enactments of problem-oriented themes (Papp & Imber-Black, 1996). Once aware of those patterns, therapists may discover the confining themes which prevent clients from solving their problems or gaining access to their own inner healer. When patterns that support the theme are altered, the theme will have to adjust because the altered patterns no longer support those specific meanings that support the problematic theme.

Here is an example of discovering a client theme through investigating patterns. I worked with a client whom I will call Kathy. Kathy went out of her way to micromanage everyone in her family. She spent much time checking and rechecking every activity of her family. From how her children ate their breakfasts to how her husband dressed for work, Kathy hovered over family members checking on them to ensure that everything went according to plan. Her constant micromanaging was causing much frustration and aggravation among family members who felt capable of doing things by themselves. In examining every aspect of her pattern of micromanagement, a theme began to emerge that I labeled, "Managing Others Brings Happiness." Kathy was unaware that her controlling everything in her home, to bring herself a sense of peace, was negatively impacting the household and giving her the opposite of what she wanted. To rectify the situation, she thought she needed to become even more controlling, which of course only created more of the problem.

After determining the constricting theme, I decided to utilize Kathy's desire to manage but adjust it so that it could be an asset to her family rather than a liability. I told Kathy that I really respected her desire to help her family by her management because it was a wonderful sign that she really cared for them all. Her problem, I said, was not that she was managing her family, but the problem lay in the patterns that she used to manage. We then discussed how good managers in companies manage their employees. We talked about how a good manager allows the employees to have some autonomy handling their tasks because it usually results in better performance. I emphasized that good managers appear to be happier and less stressed than other managers because they allowed some freedom for their employees. Kathy did not become defensive or argue during our discussion because I had accepted that her unconscious theme of controlling brought her happiness. I was simply creating a new theme for her to expand which could be titled, "A Better Manager." I ended our session with some recommendations for books about effective management styles and asked that she read up on how to be a more effective manager. I assured her that this would help her problem at home.

Over the next few weeks Kathy began to implement some of the principles she learned from her books. She realized that she had been wasting much of her time in the management of the home. She began to streamline her actions so that she could manage the family more effectively. Kathy began scheduling her own actions to alleviate stress on herself and her family as she managed multiple people in multiple situations.

Even though Kathy was still a little controlling, her family appeared to breathe a collective sigh of relief when she began to back away from overly focusing on small things. She found that once her systems were in place, she could relax and allow some freedom for her family to do things for themselves. In time, Kathy began to slowly relax more and to find a middle ground between extreme micromanaging and irresponsibility. Her new theme of being "A Better Manager" was more empowering but still showed her family that she cared. Kathy began to gain some of the happiness she sought.

Clients indirectly become more open to new perspectives and possibilities when they can experience their limiting themes in new and different ways. They may even begin to question their own rigid perspective of the problem when the habitual order of their experience has changed. When clients alter the predictable ways of interacting with their issues, they gain more behavioral flexibility which can allow them to rise above their problems. Since these alterations are not seen by the clients as directly addressing their problem, they are more apt to engage in pattern adjustments. There are four methods of pattern adjustment that I have found are successful in shifting clients' responses to their problematic themes. They are (1) altering *when* the patterns occur, (2) altering *where* the patterns occur, (3) altering the *duration* of the patterns, and (4) *adding to* the patterns.

1. Adjusting when patterns occur

Clients sometimes perform specific behavior patterns consistently, at a specific time of the day or in a specific situation. With close examination, clients sometimes find that their problems may also occur at one period of the day more than others. When these parameters are determined, therapists can then invite clients to experience their problems at different times or in different situations. This can lead to a situation in which clients deliberately try to induce their problem. This very deliberate action makes clients aware that they have more control over their problem than they realized.

I once worked with a client named Joe (and his family) on issues related to Joe's anger. Joe said that he just could not control his anger as he would like. His greatest challenge with his angry outbursts was when he was dealing with his immediate family who unintentionally triggered his wrath. Joe did not like losing control and becoming upset so easily with his family; however, he felt helpless in being able to stop it. Interactions with his family had become strained, and he felt very guilty after his outbursts. No matter how hard Joe seemed to try, he lost his battle with himself every time. He would explode in loud vocal outbursts and would then storm out of the house. He and his family felt powerless in trying to control the problem. The therapeutic theme that had arisen in our sessions could be called "Helpless Anger."

After fully examining Joe's situation, I determined that most of the outbursts appeared to occur during the week. Joe seemed to have very few anger outbursts on the weekends. When I pointed this out to Joe, he was genuinely perplexed as to why this was the case. I mused he was having so many outbursts during the week because he was not intentionally spreading his energy enough throughout the week. I told him that his energy was being built up too much over five days instead of the full seven days of the week, and this might explain why it exploded in the form of anger. Perhaps, I said, the intensity of his anger was due to having to release so much of it over a shorter time period. By allowing himself the full week to be angry instead of only five days, he might decrease the concentration of his wrath. As strange an explanation as it was, Joe seemed to accept it. The theme of therapy had shifted from "Helpless Anger" to a new theme of "Spreading Out the Energy."

I then recommended to Joe and his family that he intentionally try to have an anger outburst on both Saturday and Sunday of the next two weekends. I said that it was important to allow Joe enough space to be angry on the weekends so that he could dispense all his energy. Then perhaps the next week or two there would be fewer or less intense explosions. It took much convincing to get Joe and his family to agree because their only strategy (and comfort zone) was to avoid any anger issues, which rarely seemed to work. I told Joe to really allow himself to feel and notice everything related to his weekend outbursts so that the energy of the anger would pass more quickly. I advised the family to do what they normally did to trigger Joe's anger on the upcoming weekend so that Joe could get rid of the "anger" energy. I assured them that in doing so they would be helping Joe learn to relate to his anger in a different way.

Joe and his family reluctantly agreed to follow my directive for them: (a) do things that usually made Joe upset for the next two weekends, and (b) for Joe to allow himself to be angry at their actions in the usual manner. They were to discuss as a family what specific things they could do to trigger Joe's anger and who would do them.

In two weeks, Joe and his family came back to therapy to report that they had followed through on their directives and had created situations for Joe to become angry. The problem was that Joe was not getting angry! Joe had not had any anger outbursts on the weekends. Joe told me he had even intentionally tried to become angry so that he could get rid of any frustration he might be feeling, but he just could not respond the way he usually did. I pretended to be concerned that Joe had not become angry in spite of his family's attempts. I told them that obviously this anger was a stubborn emotion, and we might need Joe to intentionally become angry more often during the week. I asked Joe and his family to continue the assignment during the next two weeks.

After two weeks, Joe and his family returned to therapy to inform me that Joe had not been angry at all during the weekends, and he had even had very few angry outbursts during the week. When I asked Joe how was it possible that he was not reacting in his usual angry way during the week, Joe said that he had begun to notice how his body was feeling right before he got upset, and then he simply left the room to cool down. His family all agreed that Joe was not getting as angry as he previously did. They also had begun to relax more since he was not responding to their intentional attempts to provide triggers for his losing his temper. After another two weeks of Joe and his family working together for the purpose of making him angry, they found that Joe instead was becoming more relaxed. He still got irritated and frustrated by things, but his reactive outbursts had substantially decreased. They all decided that his overall anger had decreased so much that they did not need to come to therapy any more.

2. Altering where patterns occur

Breaks in a pattern can happen when the location of where a problem originates is changed. Certain actions and behaviors can have triggers which are tied to specific locations. When these triggers are unavailable, the pattern will have to adjust its process, or it will have to cease. When a change in the location takes place, clients will sometimes feel as if they have to consciously create the behavior that they had performed unconsciously. This new awareness of location and behavior helps to break the chain of emotions which have perpetuated the pattern.

Courtney and Andrew came to therapy in an effort to stop their rampant arguing which occurred almost daily. They had been together as a couple for more than three years. Both admitted to frequent bickering since the beginning of the relationship, but the severity of their arguments had escalated over the last year. As a result, they were losing much of the contentment in their relationship. They would start arguing, and emotions would build to a crescendo until they were practically screaming at each other. After the argument finally ended, each one would remain angry and not speak for several hours.

I determined that their arguments usually erupted in the evenings after dinner; however, the topics of the argument varied. It was obvious that each one was trying to control the other in their interactions, and so loud, intense disagreements ensued. Courtney broke down in tears saying that she wondered if Andrew was really motivated to resolve their issues. Andrew spoke up and said that he had the same concern about Courtney. He told me that he was so tired of their fighting and wondered if they could ever resolve their issues. Courtney agreed and said she feared that Andrew did not really value their relationship, to which Andrew replied he felt that it was she who did not value their relationship. The theme of therapy had become "A Relationship Not Valued."

Knowing both parties were projecting their own fears and concerns onto the other, I decided that any attempt to get Courtney and Andrew to gain insight into their behaviors would be futile. I asked them where in their home they argued the most. They replied that it was usually in the living room, but they assured me that they fought in every room of the house. Feeling that perhaps Courtney and Andrew were overgeneralizing their arguing activities, I asked them where the one space in their home where they had never argued was. They both thought for a few moments and then Andrew told me that they have never argued in the upstairs closet of the guest bedroom. Courtney agreed with Andrew's observation. I then asked them if they would be willing to do something a little different that could possibly help them in dealing with their consistent arguments. They both agreed that they would consider my directive. I then told them that they should not stop arguing because, at this point, it was not likely to happen. However, if they did start arguing, I only wanted them to argue in the upstairs guest bedroom closet. They both looked a little perplexed by my request. I explained that when they became involved in an argument with each other, they were to stop and immediately go upstairs into the guest bedroom closet and then continue their argument until it was over.

Both Courtney and Andrew said that they did not want to argue and really wanted to end their disagreements. This was the reason that they had sought therapy. I told them that I understood, but it was very important that there was some action that they could take as a couple to let each other know that each one was willing to do something different. I advised them that changing the location was a sign they could send to each other that they believed their issues could eventually be resolved. I said that moving their arguments to the upstairs closet was a metaphoric way to show a willingness to move their disagreements out of sight as we worked through their individual issues. Going into the closet to argue, I said, was a signal to each other that they valued their relationship enough to do something a little strange to make it better. I told them that things could be better if each one saw that their partner did indeed value their relationship even when things got very heated. Much to my surprise, they quickly accepted my proposal. Our theme for therapy changed from "A Relationship Not Valued" to "The Signaling of Value."

When they came to their next therapy session several weeks later, Courtney and Andrew told me that their daily arguments had practically ceased. They admitted to still becoming exasperated with each other at times, but the intense, long, and loud arguing that had permeated their home had decreased. Both parties reported that, by having to go to another location to fight, it showed them how silly some of their arguments had been. Courtney, in particular, declared that she realized that she had been holding on to unimportant little things. This caused a loss of her peace in her relationship. They had followed my directive to go to the closet for arguments for about a week, and then they began to notice that they were going upstairs to argue less and less. Andrew also appeared to be more open to new ways of communicating with Courtney, whereas he had been resistant in the previous therapy session. The change of location had shifted their pattern of automatic reactive arguing. From that point on, we worked on setting goals for more effective ways to interact and communicate.

3. Altering the duration of the patterns

Establishing how long the undesirable behavior lasts can also give important information and may help to change the patterns which created the behavior. Clients' answers will range from "just a few moments" to "hours" or "days." Once the duration of the problematic behavior is determined, it is fairly easy to modify the pattern. The therapist can suggest that the client extend the pattern or shorten it. Clients then become aware that they can actually have some control over their behaviors leading them to a feeling of empowerment.

Nancy came to therapy to get help for her anxiety. She had short periods of what she called "anxiety fits" in which she felt overwhelmed by anxiety. She had to get up and move around in an attempt to decrease her emotions. She became very fearful, agitated, and unable to focus her mind on anything during these anxiety fits. This had begun to cause problems for her at work when she abruptly left her desk and walked up and down the hallways to soothe her anxiety. Her boss tried to be understanding, but he was becoming frustrated when Nancy left her work space several times throughout the day. Nancy said that she had no idea why she was becoming so nervous and emotional. She felt as if she had no control over her emotions and had begun to worry that she would not be able to keep her job. She noted that she also experienced these issues when she was at home as well. Nancy had tried to solve her problem by meditation and relaxation classes in an effort to calm herself down. Unfortunately, these classes had not helped her very much, and she was still having to leave her desk at work when she became anxious. She was resistant to taking medication, but wondered if she would have to if therapy did not help her.

Since Nancy could not identify any trigger to her anxiety and did not respond well to the relaxation procedures she had learned, I determined that she needed to alter the pattern of how she reacted to her anxiety.

I asked Nancy how long her anxiety fits usually lasted. She was not sure, but guessed that they lasted around ten to fifteen minutes. I asked Nancy to buy a stopwatch and to use it to track how long her anxiety fits really lasted. She should write down the specific length of time that each one endured. She was to do this for the next week. Nancy agreed to monitor the length of the fits and to bring in her information to the next session.

When Nancy returned to therapy the next week, she had dutifully written down the length of time for the anxiety fits that she had experienced that week. I looked over the numbers and found that the average time for her fits was about fifteen minutes. I congratulated her on how well she had done in her record keeping. I then asked Nancy if she would be willing to extend her anxiety fits for five extra minutes when she had them. Nancy looked at me as if I were unhinged! I explained that her nervous system could need more time to release her anxiety than she had allowed. By adding five minutes to her fits, she could perhaps decrease how often they happened. Nancy accepted her assignment with a little coaxing on my part. Her acceptance of the assignment was aided by my agreement to write a letter to her boss informing him that Nancy was getting help and was diligently working on her problem. She just needed a little extra time to walk the halls during the next two weeks. Whether she was at work or at home, Nancy's assignment was to extend the length of time of her anxiety fits by five extra minutes. She was directed to continue her fits even if they had ceased. If she did not feel anxious after fifteen minutes, she still must continue her pacing and agitation until twenty minutes had passed. I assured her that by taking this action, she had a better chance of releasing all excessive anxiety so that the fits could decrease. The theme of therapy changed from "The Woman Who Had to Run Away" to "Five Extra Minutes for Release."

After several weeks Nancy returned to therapy to report that, for some reason, her anxiety fits had diminished considerably. She had been having less anxiety overall and had decreased her time away from her desk at work. She told me that she had found it very difficult to be anxious for the five extra minutes, but she persistently followed my request to do so for two weeks. By the end of the first week, Nancy had found that her anxiety, usually averaging about fifteen minutes, had actually decreased its length by five minutes. She found that in the second week, although still having an anxiety fit, her anxiety had declined by yet another five minutes in length. Her boss had mentioned that Nancy's time away from her desk had decreased, which was a relief to Nancy who had been worried about keeping her job. Over the next two months, Nancy continued to try to add more time to her anxiety fits, but she found that she was only being anxious for a couple of minutes. She was now better able to manage without the frequent trips away from her desk.

4. Adding to the patterns

When clients appear unable to terminate or interrupt any part of their problem, therapists can use their behavior and simply add another element to the pattern. Therapists can direct their clients to continue their present pattern, but then provide them with extra action to take. There is then no struggle with clients as they continue their undesired actions. The therapist will encourage the continuation of the action (as long as it is not physically detrimental) with the inclusion of something new. Insistence on the part of the therapist to continue the behavior is paradoxical, and in itself may make the behavior slightly different. There is less client reluctance to add another action to their patterns since the therapist does not insist on their giving up entrenched patterns. Rather than attempting to work with the clients' problems in their entirety, therapists may only need to address one part of the problem. Since they are working with only one aspect, clients feel less overwhelmed and are more open to directly addressing the problem. By adding to the problematic pattern, therapists can loosen the rigidity of the behavior. By disrupting the flow of the pattern, clients feel that they have space to adjust their previously fixed actions.

I once worked with a man whom I will call Tony who sought help for what he described as his "obsessive compulsive tendencies." He told me that he had a compulsion to touch the light switch eleven times after he turned on a light every time that he entered a room. He said that he had always been a little compulsive about things, but since he started having to touch light switches so many times, he had become more worried. When he walked into a room, he began to feel an intense sense of anxiety. If he did not touch the light switch immediately, he would become overwhelmed with panic until he finally touched it. He had to perform the task fairly quickly so that he would not be consumed by his fear. He worried that something horrible would happen if he did not perform the compulsive task of touching the light switch repeatedly. These intrusive thoughts would overpower him, and he felt helpless to stop his irrational behavior.

Tony was frustrated for not being able to stop touching the light switches. He also feared ridicule from others if they found out that he took such odd actions. He did not have the problem at work because the lights were already on, so he did not have to deal with his fear during the day. At home, however, he left most of the lights on to avoid having to constantly touch light switches. Tony worried about visiting other people's homes in case he had to turn on a light. He was exasperated with himself for feeling so out of control and being unable to cease what he clearly saw as illogical behavior. Tony was locked into a theme he had labeled as "Obsessive Compulsive Tendencies," and his frustration with himself was only making matters worse.

I complimented Tony on his valiant attempts to try to stop his tendencies. Even though he had not been successful in eliminating his problem, I believed that it was important to let him know that he had shown a dedication to get better. Even though he was not successful, his efforts were to be applauded. I then asked Tony if he would be willing to do something a little bizarre that might help his problem with light switches and anxiety. Tony said that he was open to anything that would stop his fear. With his commitment to change, I told him that the solution to his problem was that he had to "shake things up." I asked Tony to turn off the lights in his house when he was not using them. For the next two weeks every time he went into a room in his home, he was to perform his usual obsessive ritual of turning on the light, and then touching the light switch eleven times. However, now I wanted him to add something new to his pattern of behavior. For the next two weeks, when Tony entered a room and turned on a light, he was to take a new action in-between each of the eleven times he touched the light switch. This new action was to shake his whole body for a moment, then squat down and stand up, followed by slapping each of his shoulders twice with the opposite hand. If he touched the light eleven times, then he would take this action in between each of the eleven touches.

Tony agreed with my original assessment of the task that it was bizarre, but without too much convincing he agreed to take on this new task for two weeks. Since Tony lived alone and his problem primarily took place in the privacy of his own home, Tony did not feel too worried that he would appear crazy to other people. I made sure that he understood the new pattern, and I had him physically demonstrate twice what I wanted him to do before leaving my office. For the next two weeks, Tony had to leave his lights at home off all the time and take a new action in his obsessive behavior when he turned on a light.

At his next session two weeks later, Tony told me that he had followed my request and found that he was responding a little differently at home. He still felt a sense of anxiety when he entered a room and turned on a light, but he had scaled back on how many times he needed to touch the light. He said that he was now only touching the light eight times to decrease his anxiety. I told him how proud I was of his following through on his therapeutic directive. Since he had some small success from the past two weeks, I said that it was crucial that he continue his directive. This time, though, I asked him to add another piece to his pattern. I wanted him to continue the body shake, the squat, and the slapping of each shoulder twice, but he should add two slaps to each knee. He was to continue taking this bizarre action whenever he felt that he had to touch the light switch. Tony agreed and departed for another two weeks to continue his assignment now with the addition of two knee slaps. He was moving out of his theme of "Obsessive Compulsive Tendencies" and into a new theme of "Shaking Things Up."

When Tony returned two weeks later, he told me that he had again performed the task as requested, but he was now touching the light switch only three times instead of eleven. He also remarked that even though he still felt some anxiety, he didn't seem to be as frightened as he was previously. With a big smile, he told me that one day when he was in a hurry to leave for work, he realized that he had not been aware of anxiety in that moment. After another round of two weeks of squatting and slapping his shoulders and knees, Tony said that he did not feel much anxiety at all when he entered a darkened room. If he did feel anxious after turning on the light, only one or two touches to the light switch were needed. Compared to the eleven touches, only one or two touches was a huge victory for Tony who felt that he had conquered his problem.

Pattern alterations can be applied with little resistance from clients as long as therapists: (a) ensure they thoroughly understand the specific processes that clients use to sustain their problems, and (b) have a good rapport with clients so that any requests that may initially feel strange or bizarre to them will be accepted. When there is a strong therapeutic alliance, clients understand that their therapists are actively working in their best interests, and they are more likely to try new behaviors that may initially appear nonrational.

Therapeutic rituals

Extensive searching for the etiology of clients' problems and the quest for intellectual insight is often insufficient in moving clients out of problem-oriented themes. However, a task or ritual can create an experience that aids clients in relating to their problems in new and different ways. Therapeutic rituals are created for clients to represent their problems in an indirect and symbolic manner to their unconscious minds. Rituals can include any behavior, any setting, or element that can express the problem situation in a tangible way. This allows clients to indirectly work through and transcend their particular problem in a manner that is unique to them. These rituals can help produce changes in the clients' emotional and cognitive patterns using their own ability to unconsciously generate healing in a manner not provided by consciously oriented interventions (Van Der Hart, 1983). Therapeutic rituals have been used to "facilitate client change, restore connectedness to community and higher powers, and create a sense of structure" (Crockett & Prosek, 2013, p. 242).

The purpose of introducing therapeutic rituals into therapy sessions is to provide clients with tasks that open avenues to increased flexibility and access to their own internal resources. When clients perform the designated ritual, they have experience of dealing with their problem in a totally different way. It also adds a random element to their experience. Clients unconsciously benefit from more possibilities in how they respond to their situation. The performance of therapeutic theme-related rituals allows the patterns and meanings of those themes to become obvious and dramatized. As Papp and Imber-Black (1996) suggest, "[S]ymbolizing the theme … is a particularly effective way to expand the conversation" (p. 16).

Rituals can be mysterious since many ritual meanings are often hidden or not easily discerned by the participants. Almost every culture has had rituals in order to evoke protection, social order, or access to the supernatural. These practices are historically transmitted generationally and may be openly shared, or they may be kept secret by the participants. Ritualistic practices may take the form of particular prayers, the use of charms, specific movements and dances, or individualized quests. Each culture has its own perspective on how rituals are to be performed and also when to perform them. These rituals are usually not random and, even though they may be distinctive in many ways, there are more similarities than differences between them in the process in which they are constructed and the psychological aspects that are involved (Goodwyn, 2016).

Human nature seems to intuitively seek to connect with something more mysterious, and rituals allow participants to contact those mysterious parts of themselves. Ritual actions are much more than "a repetitive behavior or activity; rather, they give meaning to individuals' experiences through the active use of symbols, which parallel the experiences of individuals with a power greater than themselves" (Crockett & Prosek, 2013, p. 241). Rituals can increase the awareness of the formerly unconscious aspects of participants, can alter their consciousness, and can provide them with meaning in situations where meaning was previously absent.

Crockett and Prosek (2013) define rituals as a distinctive set of characteristics which include "universality, the facilitation of transitions and change, the mobilization of supernatural powers, the creation of new meaning, and the formation of a new identity" (p. 240). Cole (2003) found that three changes promoted by rituals are: (1) adjustments in psychological state, (2) transitions in significant phases of life, and (3) connections in emotional and relational realms. Rituals can help clients who have used intellectual insight to try to change their emotions and perceptions but with limited results. These activities "offer clients the opportunity to create a space through a structured intervention that works to promote client wellness, while restoring a sense of order and security in life" (Crockett & Prosek, 2013, p. 242).

When clients are provided with an out-of-the-ordinary and mystifying experience, they are required to go beyond their cognitive efforts in dealing with their problematic situations. Mysterious and strange experiences can bypass the clients' conscious thinking processes and reach them at a deeper unconscious level which can guide them to a more flexible response to their problem. As Goodwyn (2016) points out, "The brain plays a fundamental part in ritual experience through its capacity to co-create a cognized and highly symbolic world" (p. 26). Participation in rituals has been shown to activate the autonomic nervous system in a way that can both stimulate and calm subcortical neural processing which leads to increased emotional connection (Hogue, 2006). Rituals that possess powerful symbolism and produce intense emotional experiences can lead to an increased right-brain processing that may lead to shifts in personal perspectives (Goodwyn, 2016).

The construction of therapeutic rituals can be built around the analogies and metaphors that clients use to describe their situations. A remarkable amount of information about the clients' perceptions and distinctions about their problems can be found in their own descriptive phrases. Some phrases used by clients to describe their situations such as "my back is against the wall," "stuck in a rut," "frozen in time," "pulled in too many directions," or "between a rock and a hard place," can provide therapists with ideas for tasks and rituals which reach clients at their unconscious level. These metaphors give therapists a map of what resources the clients may connect to and what specific rituals can create those connections. By using these metaphors to create ritual actions, therapists help clients in building a bridge to new themes that enhance their lives. As Kirmayer (1993) states,

> Metaphoric constructions are not final but tentative; they do not always reflect an underlying representation or even preverbal body-knowing but are a sallying forth, a presentation of what is possible and hence, the invention of a potential truth to which we may commit ourselves to varying degrees. (p. 185)

Once we notice the metaphors that clients use to describe their problem, we can designate a symbolic action corresponding to their metaphor. We then can direct clients to take this uncommon action involving the assigned symbol to interrupt the patterns of their unconscious themes. This symbolic ritual must require some effort on the part of clients, or it will not have the emotional impact needed to create change. For example, if a client says that she feels "tied to her past," she may be directed to pick a color that represents her past and then to paint a rope with that color. She would then be directed to tie herself up with the painted rope, now the symbolic color of her past, and stay tied up for three hours. She would then untie herself and burn the rope. This symbolic act moves the client from her problem theme of "Tied to the Past" to a new theme of "The Escape Artist." By using the metaphors that clients articulate, new tasks and rituals can be produced to create change at the unconscious, symbolic level.

Norman came to see me because of the many changes that he had experienced over the past two years. He had lost his job and changed careers. He was divorced, lost his mother to cancer, and moved to a new town. He had also turned fifty years old and was beginning to feel his age with some issues with his back. Norman told me that his mother's death had hit him hard. She had rapidly deteriorated not long after receiving her diagnosis of cancer. Norman saw parallels between his mother's quick death and the quick ending of his marriage, his necessary change of career, and relocation. He was having trouble accepting the many changes in his life, and he longed to return to his way of life before the last two years. Even though Norman knew that going back in time was an impossibility, he found that he fantasized too much about how things used to be. He had become depressed in his present life. Consciously, Norman was well aware that he needed to focus on his current life and to direct himself toward new goals. He knew he must accept the reality of his situation; however, he just could not get himself to move beyond the unconscious blocks that continued to freeze him in his past.

After working with Norman for a couple of sessions, it became very obvious that he was unable to accept where he was in his life. He frequently told me that he wished he could just "bury his past" and focus on his future, but he felt he was a prisoner of his past. Norman reported that he frequently dreamed about his old life and would then wake up disappointed that it had only been a dream. Even though he was fully aware of his limiting beliefs about his life, he still seemed unable to shake the feelings he was experiencing. All attempts at cognitive restructuring went nowhere. Norman was very conscious of his thinking patterns, and he did his best to dispute the constraining patterns in his thinking but to little avail. Norman was locked in a disempowering theme of "Living in the Past." I decided that the only way to shift Norman out of his fixed patterns of thought and emotion was to give him a therapeutic ritual symbolizing his problem. Hopefully this would help him access his inner resources and he could move forward in his life. I hoped that Norman was up to the task that I devised for him.

    I asked Norman to come up with a color that represented his old life. He thought for a moment and then said that his old life would be best represented by a dark green. He chose this color because he thought green was a pleasant color; but because his past was something that he wanted to be free from, it had to be a darker color to represent the negative aspects of it. Norman had said in an earlier session that he enjoyed doing small woodworking projects so I decided to incorporate his hobby into his therapeutic ritual. I asked Norman to build a small wooden box with any leftover wood that he might have. After building the box, Norman was to paint the box the dark green color he had chosen to represent his old life. He was then to find one important item from each area of his past life that had been very important to him. He was to find an item related to his mother, his marriage, his old job, and where he used to live. He was to put all of these items into his newly built wooden box. After filling the box, he was to take it to a local forest and find a secluded, hidden area in which he could bury the box. Since Norman had frequently used the metaphor of "bury the past," I believed that he needed a symbolic action that responded to that desire. Norman was to leave the box in the ground for a whole week. After that time, he would then retrieve it from the forest.

    With much persuasion on my part, Norman agreed to take on this ritual. He returned home, built his box, and painted it dark green. For the items to go into the box, he chose a tie he had worn often at his old job, a copy of his wedding picture, a T-shirt with a logo of a restaurant he used to frequent in his former town, and a hairbrush that used to belong to his mother. Norman picked a time late in the evening when few people were visiting the forest. He found an out-of-the-way location, dug a hole, and place his box in it. He buried the box and quickly left the area. A week later he came back to the forest and retrieved his buried box filled with representations of his old life.

When Norman came back to see me after he had completed his ritual, he told me how surprisingly difficult the task had been for him. He expressed how emotional he had become when he was putting the items into the box and then burying them in the earth. Norman disclosed that he experienced very vivid dreams about his ex-wife the night after he buried his box. He also said that he was not able to concentrate much for a couple of days after he buried his "old life." By the time a week had passed, however, Norman found that he was thinking a little less about his old life than he usually did. He revealed that when he dug up his box and took it home, he avoided taking the items out of the box for a day. When he finally opened it and took the items out, they felt different to him and did not seem to have the same emotional charge they previously possessed. Norman even noted that the night he opened the box, he had had a dream about his mother that was quite comforting, which was different from his earlier dreams about her passing. It appeared that Norman's unconscious was letting him know that it was time for him to begin moving forward. He even told me that he felt he was finally "getting the signal" to start a new phase in his life. Therapy progressed much easier when the theme of the sessions changed from "Living in the Past" to "Getting the Signal." Norman found that, even though he missed some things about his old life, he was more open to new possibilities for his future.

* * *

When we bypass our etiology-oriented conversations and shift to pattern alterations, metaphoric tasks, and symbolic rituals, we can help our clients to break out of their "problem-entrenched" themes. If we are to be effective with these interventions, we must be creative and be willing to venture into the unknown domain of the clients' unconscious minds. We must focus more attention on how our clients perform and represent their problems with less attention on "why" they have the problems. When we do this, we have more options as we and our clients cocreate more hopeful and affirmative themes.

CHAPTER 5

The soldier who was secretly a hippie

This session was with Amber, a forty-five-year-old woman. She came to her session conservatively dressed, but also had a streak of the color green in her hair which she was wearing in a ponytail. On her paperwork she listed the presenting problem to be "issues with coping."

[C = Client | T = Therapist]

T: How can I help you today?
C: I am a little nervous. I have never had a male therapist.
T: I see. You have been in therapy previously?
C: Yes sir. I went to a couple of different therapists over the past eight years. I had problems with alcohol and had to go to rehab. They had some therapists at the facility and I was encouraged to continue seeing someone for therapy after I left the outpatient part of the program. All of the therapists were female so it is just a little different. I mean, it's fine you're a man. I guess I just don't know what to expect.
T: I understand. What was your experience like with the other therapists?

(I always ask how clients' previous experiences of therapy were because if something the other therapists did worked, I want to utilize what has been successful. If, however, things previous therapists did with clients didn't work, then I want to avoid doing similar actions.)

C: They were good. I went for a while and then I would quit. I would then go back when I needed to go back. They were all very nice and helpful. They allowed me to talk and figure things out.
T: I am glad to hear that. You mentioned that you had a problem with alcohol. Are things better for you now?
C: Yes sir. I attend regular Alcoholics Anonymous meetings and I have a sponsor. That has helped. I realized that I had been uncomfortable feeling bad feelings so I would move to drink to distract myself. There were also issues with back pain which probably caused me to drink more than I should because it decreased some of the pain.
T: How long have you had the back pain?
C: For over fifteen years. I was in a vehicle accident when I was in the Army and I had some really bad problems with my back. I've had two back surgeries which have helped a little, but my pain still bothers me. My accident was the reason I left the Army.
T: How long were you in the Army?
C: I was in for close to eight years.
T: Did you like being in the Army?
C: Yes sir. I did. Now, to be honest, it was tough going into the Army as a woman, but in time some things eased up. The Army gave me some structure which I needed at that time. I had some good friends and didn't get stationed too terribly far from home. When I hurt my back, the Army retired me out. Since I have back trouble I can only work for a few hours a week so I am happy to get a little bit of money from the military. My husband has a good job so we get by. But, yes sir, I enjoyed being in the Army.
T: That's great. It sounds like you still are in the Army because you keep saying "Yes sir."
C: [*Laughs*] Yeah, I was also brought up to say that.
T: I was too.
C: Sometimes I kind of miss the Army, but at the same time I enjoy having my own schedule and doing things I enjoy. The back pain still

bothers me. I was on pain medication for a while. It really wasn't helping that much. I was also on antidepressant medication and something for anxiety. My psychiatrist initially thought I might have been cyclothymic, but now he thinks I am just having issues with depression and anxiety. I stopped taking the pain medication six months ago because it was causing me to feel weird and mentally numb. Please don't tell anyone, but I smoke marijuana in the mornings. Since I started smoking my pain has really decreased and I don't feel like I am numb or anything. I get up in the morning and smoke and then an hour or so later I feel fine. I guess I am silly saying for you not to tell anyone. I know these sessions are confidential. I guess I just don't want people I know to find out. I go to church and am very active in my church community.

T: I don't think you are being silly to worry about confidentiality.
C: [*Laughs*] OK.
T: You mentioned your church. Are you a religious person?
C: Yes sir. I am very religious. I think God has helped me through many of my trials in life.
T: OK. It sounds like people in your church are important to you.
C: Yes sir. They are. None of them know that I had to go to rehab years ago. Maybe I should tell them? I don't know.
T: How long have you been dealing with depression and anxiety?
C: For close to fifteen years.
T: Around the time of your accident?
C: Yes sir. Believe it or not, the marijuana has helped my anxiety a little.
T: OK.
C: I think if I didn't have pain, I might not smoke it every day, but it helps.
T: I understand. Well, let me ask you, what specifically motivated you to come see me today?
C: I have been having a personal issue that I just don't know how to deal with and it's causing me so much turmoil. I just don't know how to say it to anyone. I have only told one other person about it.
T: Who was the person you told?
C: My best friend, Elaine.
T: You must really trust Elaine.
C: Yes sir, I do. She has been with me through so much over the past ten years.

T: It's good to have people you trust in your life.

C: I just don't know how to say it other than just say it. [*Begins to cry*] I have been having an affair for close to a year. It's with a man who I have known since I was a teenager … he and I were friends for a few years. [*Amber stops to cry for a few moments*] It just happened and I … don't seem to be able to stop it. I am so ashamed. I know better but yet, I keep doing it. I want to stop, but I just can't seem to stop. I'm sorry … [*Begins crying again*]

T: That's OK. This secret must have been pretty tough for you to carry for so long.

C: It is.

T: Tell me how this all started.

C: This man, his name is Mark, and I knew each other when I was younger … back in high school. It was just two friends, nothing else. I graduated and left for the Army and I never talked to him until about two years ago. I ran into him at the grocery store and we started talking again. For close to a year nothing happened between us, but one day I went over to see him at his house and we ended up going too far. He's divorced. It is like he has this power over me now. It seems like I can't stop talking to him and going to see him. When he asks me to come over, I can't seem to say no to him. Elaine tells me that Mark is toxic for me, but I keep going back. I love my husband … and want to be faithful … [*Begins to cry again*] … I just can't seem to stop myself.

T: What is your husband's name?

C: Karl.

T: So Karl has no idea …

C: No sir. He doesn't. He works long days and sometime is out of town for his job during the day. He's a good man. A really good man. I just hate that … I keep doing this. I just hate it. I don't know what's wrong with me. I am just so ashamed of myself. We were married in the eyes of God and in the church, and then I go and do this. [*Continues crying for a few moments*]

T: So you have been hiding this secret and it has been tough to conceal it.

C: Yes sir. I can't sleep much because I keep running through my head all the things I know I shouldn't be doing, but I keep doing. I have lost about twenty pounds over the past few months. I have not felt like eating like I know I need to because I think I am just so worked up about this …

T: Yeah.

C: … situation I am in. I feel like my brain is just not working right.

T: How long have you been married?

C: Almost fifteen years.

T: Do you have any children?

C: We have one son, Jimmy. He is from a previous relationship. Karl has been his father though. Jimmy is twenty years old. He's away at college now. We see him maybe every other month for a weekend.

T: So Jimmy isn't around much.

C: No.

T: OK. Other than this situation, how is your marriage? Do you feel like it …

C: It's good. I mean he is really good to me. He doesn't have an issue with me not working much because of my back. He doesn't mistreat me. He totally lets me do my artwork all over the house. He is such a nice guy. I am really torn up at what is going on … [*Crying*] … He just deserves better … a lot better.

T: I'm really sorry to hear you are going through this situation.

C: I just can't stop with Mark. I feel so stuck and helpless. I know I shouldn't talk to him, but I do. I know I shouldn't go see him, but I do. I'm just … I'm just crazy or something. I'm afraid my family will find out and I don't know if I could bear the shame of it … I just don't know.

(Amber has a fully developed theme that I will call "The Woman Who Wants to Be Good, But Is Bad." It is obvious to me that she is emotionally beating herself up due to this secret she has been carrying. As long as we stay rooted in her theme of her being "bad," any intervention may be more fuel for her thoughts about her being bad.)

T: I know this is tough for you. May I ask what have you previously done to change this situation?

C: I tried not talking to Mark, but I would end up calling him after a few days.

T: OK. So not calling did not seem to help when you tried it?
C: No sir. I really didn't want to call, but I just found myself doing it. I would end up calling and then going over to see him. On the way back home I would hate myself.
T: I see. You mentioned telling your friend …
C: Elaine.
T: Yes, Elaine. What did she tell you about this problem?
C: She said Mark was really just using me. She said he was toxic for me and would end up destroying what I have with Karl. She just can't seem to understand why I keep doing it. I can't either.
T: Did Elaine tell you anything that has helped you with Mark?
C: No. She is just supportive of me, but she is worried that I will continue this mess until things fall apart.
T: OK.
C: I love my husband, but Mark just seems to give me something I can't let go of … he has a hold on me. When my husband and I make love it's nice, but it's just … a little boring. With Mark it is like he unleashes something in me. I feel things I haven't felt much with Karl.
T: Do you feel that sex is the primary motivation to see Mark?
C: I don't want to admit it, but it is. I like Mark and he makes me laugh, but if I had to be honest with you, I would have to say that sex is probably the main thing. That sounds so terrible …
T: It's fine. You are just being honest.
C: I know, but I hate to hear myself say that.
T: I understand. Do you think there is ever a possibility that you could share this with your husband? I mean …
C: No sir! I would rather die than tell him. He has been so good to me. I don't know if I could live with myself if I had to tell him about Mark.
T: I see.
C: Mark just brings out things in me that Karl doesn't. He is open to things I am afraid to approach Karl with … it is just different. I really don't know …
T: If Karl was more open to you in those ways, do you think Mark would be so interesting?
C: I don't know. I doubt I would feel as trapped as I am. Maybe if Karl and I had a different relationship in that area, maybe I wouldn't.

T: Have you talked with Karl about seeking marital counseling?
C: No. I'm too afraid the whole stuff with Mark would come out so I don't want to do that.
T: So, just so I understand, if Karl was more open sexually with you, then Mark might not hold as much interest to you?
C: Yes sir, probably. It's not like anything is bad with Karl, he just … he just doesn't take things as seriously or intensely when we make love. He laughs a lot and acts silly. I don't guess there is anything wrong with that, but it keeps me from wanting to have more intense moments with him.
T: And have you directly discussed the lack of intensity with Karl?
C: Not really … I think it would hurt his feelings and cause us problems.
T: Problems?
C: I mean that he might start doubting himself and it would affect our intimate time together.
T: Oh. So you are saying that your concern for his feelings has stopped you from talking about this with him?
C: Yes … it's also uncomfortable to talk about I guess … it's just so personal.
T: I get that.
C: I want to let Mark go, but I can't seem to do it. Every time after I see him I swear that I won't see him again and the next thing that I know, I am driving over to see him. Like I said, it is like he has some hold on me.
T: Have you talked with Mark about how you are feeling about seeing him?
C: I tried to once on the phone, but he didn't seem to care much …
T: He didn't care about what you were saying?
C: No. He just kind of brushed off my comments.
T: So he doesn't care about what this is doing to you?
C: I don't think so.
T: That doesn't sound too kind to me.
C: I guess it isn't. In some ways I am mad at Mark because he knows how it destroys me and doesn't seem to care, but yet I want to keep seeing him.
T: If Mark suddenly said that he didn't want to see you anymore, would it …

C: It would help me. If he moved on and left me alone. I think I could just focus on other things.
T: I see. If he lost interest, then you could move on?
C: Yes sir. I sometimes wish he would.
T: You mentioned being able to focus on other things. What specific other things?
C: I'm sorry, I don't follow ...
T: What other things would you be focusing on if this situation with Mark was not going on?
C: I would probably do more of my artwork ...
T: Yeah, you mentioned Karl is fine with you doing your artwork all over the house.
C: Yes sir. He actually likes it.
T: What kind of artwork do you like to do?
C: I love to paint. I will paint pictures of landscapes. I also paint different things, like lamps or furniture. You should see my house, in one room it is filled with furniture of all kinds of wild colors. I painted the two tables in the room bright reds and oranges and the lamps are bright green. It is just a ton of color.
T: Like a tie-dyed room?
C: [*Laughs*] Yes, it is full of different bright colors. I didn't think Karl would like it, but he does.
T: Are the other rooms in the house also that colorful?
C: No, the other rooms are painted in more subdued colors. It looks different. I like for there to be differences in the house.
T: OK. What else do you paint?
C: I wish I could paint people, but I have never been good at that. I like to paint nature. I will see a pretty landscape photo in a magazine and I will try to paint it. Sometimes I can get close to how the photo looks, but other times I just get too creative and embellish it. A few months ago I did a painting of this waterfall and halfway through the painting I decided to add some more trees and rocks than what was in the painting.
T: That sounds like you are a very creative person.
C: I don't know. I just like to draw and paint. I guess it relaxes me.
T: When was the last time you painted?
C: I don't know ... maybe four months ago.

T: That sounds like a really long time for someone who is creative.
C: It is, but with all that is going on, I can't get myself to do anything. I want to draw, but my mind is just spinning so much … I can't focus.
T: I think you need to get back into your art.
C: I know. I just don't know where to start.
T: What other things do you do for enjoyment when you aren't worrying about this situation?
C: I like to garden.
T: Really?
C: Oh yes! I have a small garden behind our house where I plant vegetables.
T: What kind of vegetables?
C: Things like tomatoes, peas, squash, corn … a lot of those kind of things. I also like to plant flowers and decorative bushes around the house. It gets me outside and I can mix and match different colors.
T: Kind of like art?
C: Yes, like art. I guess it is doing art with the color and all …
T: When was the last time you got out in the garden?
C: It has been a couple of weeks. The tomatoes are still growing. I have to make sure they don't get too much water. I planted some begonias around the back of the house. They look really pretty. I need to plant some bluebells back there, but I don't know if the soil is good enough.
T: You really get into gardening, don't you?
C: [*Laughs*] Yes sir. I enjoy it. I am always learning new things about plants. I just like being out in nature. I really enjoy just sitting out in the woods behind our home. It helps me calm down a little. It's quiet and no one bothers me.
T: How often do you do that?
C: I try to do it fairly often.
T: Do you cook with your vegetables?
C: Oh yes! I try to cook really healthy foods for us. I like to avoid any processed foods and eat as natural as possible. I have been learning about how to avoid those things in our meals. I am also learning about cooking gluten free.
T: I see. Does Karl like your cooking?
C: He does. He tries to help me in the kitchen sometimes.

(At this point, I have heard enough new information to start moving Amber into a new theme for the session.)

T: Listen, I don't mean to change the subject, but something has just occurred to me.
C: What?
T: I think you may be a hippie!
C: [*Laughs*] What?
T: No, really. It sounds like you are a hippie.
C: Why do you say that?
T: Well, you seem to really enjoy interacting with nature, you are into different kinds of art, you believe in eating as naturally as possible, you smoke pot, and you have a green streak of color in your hair. I mean, think about it … even one of the rooms in your home is a "tie-dyed" room.
C: [*Laughs*] I guess in a way I am …
T: And here is the thing, you are not just a hippie, you are a soldier who is secretly a hippie. It is like you are living in two worlds: the military world and the hippie world.
C: I haven't thought about that …
T: And it may be that you have to keep some of that hippie in you secret because some people might not understand. For example, some of the people in your church might not understand having a multicolored room or a pot-smoking, gardening artist.
C: Yeah.
T: Some people that you may know in your community just might not understand eating off their own land or creating really wild artwork.
C: That's true.
T: You have been hiding this secret from many people. There is nothing wrong with you being a secret hippie, it just might not be something that you wanted to share with everyone.
C: I haven't thought about it that way.
T: Yeah, on the outside we have Amber of the Army that follows the traditional rules, and then we have Amber the Hippie who is a free spirit and is just trying to do things she enjoys. She is into peace and love and doing creative things. I think it is very cool!
C: Yeah, I see that.

(Amber has now started to buy into the new theme of the session: "The Soldier That Was Secretly a Hippie." From this new theme, resources such as being creative and artistic can be employed to help Amber.)

T: OK, here is a serious question for you. Are you ready to hear it?
C: What?
T: Does Karl know that he is married to a soldier who is secretly a hippie?
C: [*Laughs*] I don't know. He's never called me a hippie.
T: So would it be surprising to him to learn you are a hippie?
C: Probably not. He sees all my artwork and puts up with it.
T: Sure. What if you were to go home and tell him? You know, go home and just say, "Karl, I have a confession to make, I am really a hippie." What would he say?
C: [*Laughs*] I don't know. He would probably be like, "OK honey." [*Laughs*]
T: Yeah, so he could handle the secret.
C: I guess so.
T: You know, what is really coming up for me as we are talking is that I think some of your problem is due to you not being authentic with who you are with Karl.
C: What do you mean?
T: I think that you kind of want to live the hippie lifestyle, but maybe you don't really want to come out about it or maybe you don't want to do it alone. Look at how you are living in two worlds. You are dressed really nicely, but there is that artistic streak with the green in your hair. I think that perhaps you just need to be able to be more yourself when you are at home with Karl.
C: He knows that I do art and that I garden … and the pot.
T: Yeah. But have you ever thought about what it would be like to be totally open about being a secret hippie at home?
C: I never thought about it.
T: Of course not. This is a secret that you have not really thought about.
C: So I need to tell Karl?
T: Maybe, I think you could consider telling Karl that even though you are going to be a soldier in public, at home you are going to be a total hippie. Here is the thing, I think he may need to open up a little to your hippie side.

C: How do you mean?

T: If you come out fully as a hippie to Karl, then there can be no expectation that you will be a soldier at home. He may have to become a little more flexible with you. I predict that if you really let your creative and artsy side run wild, you may have to make sure that Karl can roll with the punches. You may have to help him loosen up a little. I remember you telling me that you didn't think he would like the way you painted some furniture, but he ended up liking it. He may have to open up more …

C: Because of all the art …

T: Art and nature. You are really holistic in your cooking and health, right?

C: I try to be.

T: Sure. You two may find that you may have a little more freedom if you both start to explore the hippie side.

C: What would he have to do?

T: I'm not sure, he will have to figure out the best way to roll with the punches. He may be totally open to it, or he may feel threatened by it, or …

C: I don't think he will be threatened by it. He is really supportive of the things I like to do.

T: Great! Do you think you could tell him that you have been holding back on how much you are a hippie and into nature and health … art, you know? And just tell him that you want to be more yourself and open about it more at home.

C: I could.

T: Great. I know this is not why you came to see me, but I think it is important to your mental state. Being able to be more open about who you are with your loved ones can only help you feel more comfortable at home … maybe you could use a little more comfort lately?

C: [*Laughs*] I certainly could!

T: Just think about it. What would be the first hippie thing you could do after you tell Karl about being a hippie that will surprise him and let him know that you are really serious?

C: Hmmm … I guess I could finish painting the nightstand in our room some crazy colors.

T: Nice!

C: I could make it look a little wild.
T: What would Karl think?
C: Probably not much. I think he is used to my wild colors.
T: You know what? I think we need to get Karl into the spirit of things. Does he have a tie-dyed shirt?
C: I don't think so.
T: Could you buy him a tie-dye shirt to wear?
C: I guess I could. I don't think I have ever seen him with one.
T: Listen, this is going to sound really crazy, OK. I know this will sound a little silly, but I am very serious about it. Can I tell you my thought?
C: Yes sir.
T: I think you should plan a secret party for you and Karl to celebrate your hippie union.
C: A party?
T: Yeah, with balloons and a tie-dye cake. You could get the bakery to make it special. I think you could wrap up a tie-dye shirt as a gift for Karl. He could come home from work one evening and you can have a surprise party for you two going the way of the hippie.
C: That's crazy! I like it though. I could get different color balloons. I could make an outfit that looks like the 1960s hippies that I could wear to surprise him.
T: I love it! Yeah …
C: And I could get him some beads to wear and give him his shirt.
T: Yeah, you could make it like a performance art piece. You could call it "The Age of Aquarius and Amber." You could really surprise him!
C: [*Laughs*] This is really silly.
T: It absolutely is. Will you do it?
C: I'll do it. Should I invite anyone else?
T: It is up to you. You could just invite people you trust, like your friend Elaine, or you could just have it for the two of you. Whatever you think is best.
C: I think I will just have it for me and Karl. [*Laughs*] He might think I have gone off the deep end.
T: He may.
C: Probably not. He's a good sport.
T: OK. Will you do this for me? Will you plan this party within the next week?

C: Yes sir.
T: I think this is really important to be open with Karl about who you are. It seems silly, but you may be amazed how this can help.
C: I'll do it. I could probably plan it for this Friday. Karl doesn't work this weekend so we could just spend Friday evening doing the party.
T: Can you get him a tie-dye shirt by then?
C: Yes, I can actually pick it up this afternoon.
T: Excellent! I love it.

Amber left the session stating she was headed to the store to buy the tie-dyed shirt for Karl. Amber returned to therapy three weeks later. She stated that she had decorated her home for the party and surprised Karl who thought the party idea was hilarious. They both enjoyed the cake and Karl liked his new tie-dye t-shirt. Amber also told me that, over the past three weeks, she and Karl had become a little closer and talking more. She stated that they had been having sex more often and Karl was acting more serious and passionate when they were making love. Amber also revealed that she had not visited Mark at all since her last session. She did state that she had talked to him a few times on the phone, but she had not gone over to see him. She was both puzzled and empowered by her lack of engaging with Mark. On her third session several weeks later, Amber stated that she was asking Karl more directly for what she wanted when they made love and told me that she felt much closer to him. She also stated that she had only talked to Mark once on the phone and did not feel the impulsive pull to see him anymore. Amber beamed as she showed me pictures of all her new artwork and gardening which was keeping her very busy as of late. I also noticed that, in addition to the streak of green in her hair, there was also a streak of red. Amber was still a soldier, but her hippie side really seemed to be enjoying itself.

CHAPTER 6

The heart of an artist

This session took place at an outpatient clinic. It was with Miriam, a twenty-year-old woman, who came to therapy with a presenting complaint of feeling depressed. She had no previous history of being in therapy.

[C = Client | T = Therapist]

T: What brings you in?
C: I don't know where to begin. I am new to this kind of thing.
T: That's fine, you can begin wherever you want.
C: It's just that I am not sure what is important for you to know.
T: No worries. I will ask you to clarify if I need more info and …
C: OK.
T: … I will let you know.
C: OK.
T: Whatever you would like to discuss …
C: I guess I'm depressed. I also have a lot of anxiety. I have trouble managing my moods. I will feel better for a short time and I start feeling pulled back down into my depression. I don't want to feel that way …

T: Can you describe your depression?
C: I don't understand …
T: I mean, can you tell me what you are experiencing when you feel depressed?
C: Yeah, um, I feel a tremendous feeling of emptiness. It kind of feels like … like my body is heavy. I am not sure if that is what you mean?
T: Yes, exactly.
C: OK. I feel this feeling of emptiness and heaviness. It is like I am getting pulled down into this pit of gloom and hopelessness. I don't want to get pulled down, but I feel like I don't have a choice. I mean, it even feels heavy to walk around sometimes …
T: Yeah …
C: … because I can't seem to get out of the pit. I really want to take off the heaviness, but I feel like it is attached to me. Like it is a heavy jacket I am wearing that I can't see and that I can't take off. It is kind of like my body aches, but it doesn't physically hurt, you know, it's not like having a sharp pain …
T: Yes.
C: I just can't shake it off.
T: How long have you had this going on?
C: Probably as long as I can remember.
T: Even when you were a little child?
C: Well … no. It probably started when I was in middle school. At least that is when I remember feeling it somewhat. It seems that it wasn't as bad back then. I think it has got worse over the last year to maybe two years.
T: What have you previously done to try and cope with the feeling?
C: I used to try and distract myself. I played sports in school and that would help sometimes.
T: What sports did you play?
C: I did softball and volleyball.
T: Were you good at them?
C: I wasn't bad, but I wasn't great.
T: Are you being modest?
C: [*Laughs*] No. I just could tell that there were some other girls who had more natural ability than me.
T: Did you have fun though?

C: Yeah, for the most part. We didn't get into the finals, but we got close. My volleyball team was more fun for me. We almost made it to the finals in our region. The girls on that team were nice and we had a good time playing.
T: That's nice. Are you doing any sports now?
C: No, I am not really into that kind of thing anymore.
T: What kind of things are you into now?
C: Not much.
T: Not much? Do you mean you are not into too many things or you are not into anything?
C: Really nothing now. I haven't done much other than work and help take care of my grandmother.
T: Is you grandmother ill?
C: No, she is just becoming more limited in being able to get around so I help her with some yard work and run errands for her.
T: That is really nice of you to help her out. How old is she?
C: She is close to eighty years old.
T: I assume you are close to her.
C: I am.
T: Does she know about how you have been feeling?
C: No. She knows that some days I don't feel too active, but I have not told her that it has been getting worse. I try to only go over on days when I feel I have more energy so she doesn't notice anything.
T: You are trying to protect your grandmother from how you are feeling?
C: I just don't want her to be worried or upset.
T: Yeah, that is what I meant. You are trying to protect her from feeling bad about you feeling bad.
C: Yes. She has enough to worry about than worrying about me.
T: You put other people first a lot don't you?
C: Yes. I do that often.
T: You must be a very kind person.
C: I don't know about that, but I try to be nice to most people.
T: Do you live alone?
C: No, right now I live with my parents. I wanted to go off to college, but I decided to stay in the area and take classes at the local college to save money. My parents are fine with me living with them if I pay

for my own car insurance and contribute a little money for food. They also appreciate me helping out with grandma.
T: Because that probably helps them not have to spend so much of their time worrying and looking after her?
C: Yeah.
T: Do you get along with your parents?
C: I think so. My mother can be a little bossy sometimes. It's probably because she is a nurse.
T: [*Laughs*] Because she has to boss her patients around to get them to do what they need to do?
C: [*Laughs*] Yeah, and I think she forgets that Dad and I are not her patients sometimes.
T: That can happen.
C: But I love her. She and I get along fairly well. It's just every now and then we argue. Not much.
T: And Dad?
C: We get along well. He is always involved with different projects with his work, but we usually are fine.
T: Good. Do your parents know how you have been feeling as of late?
C: Not really, they will sometimes comment on how I don't seem like myself. They are very busy themselves so aren't home much.
T: Are you protecting them as well?
C: Maybe … I just don't want them to worry.
T: I see.
C: They would probably get really worried if I told them that I was really depressed.
T: And it would bother you that they might be worried?
C: Yeah. I wouldn't want that.
T: So it sounds like you are really just having to deal with this stuff by yourself.
C: I am. I really want to feel better, but I just have this heavy depressed feeling that consumes me sometimes. Like I said, I feel like I am wearing some heavy jacket that I can't take off. Like it is some kind of heavy iron jacket that I have to wear.
T: How have you tried to take that jacket off previously?
C: Do you mean how have I tried to deal with the depression?
T: Yes.

C: I have tried to stay busy. That can help, but sometimes I feel like I am down for several days, maybe even a week or two. I can't seem to pull myself out of it. I just don't want to go anywhere or see anyone.

T: I understand.

C: Something I haven't told anyone is that I sometimes cut myself. [*Starts to cry*]

T: I understand. Are you cutting yourself due to having to wear this iron jacket?

C: Yeah … I feel so empty inside and depressed that … [*Pauses to cry*] It happens when I get overwhelmed by the depression. I just don't want to feel it anymore. When I am in that pit of sadness … it helps me feel something else. I feel something other than the depression. I sometimes feel a little better but I just know that it's going to come back. It is like I do better but then I get pulled back into it.

T: Are you hurting yourself in other ways?

C: No. I am not intentionally trying to hurt myself or commit suicide or anything like that. It is …

T: Do you cut yourself when you are feeling better or only when you …?

C: No … and I don't cut every time I feel bad. It's just when I get overwhelmed by it all. I am ashamed about it. I haven't told anyone else …

T: You haven't told any other person about …

C: Well, I did tell a friend of mine when I first did it. I did it for the first time in high school. I only did it once or twice. I told my best friend. Her name is Jessie. She didn't tell anyone.

T: Do you still talk to Jessie?

C: Not often. She is away at college so we only really talk when she comes home on the breaks. I haven't told her about depression or cutting lately.

T: OK.

(A theme has emerged in my mind that the client is experiencing. The theme is "The Woman Who Wore an Iron Jacket." Any actions taken within this theme will maintain the duality of "good days" and "bad days." She has good days when she feels better, but she knows bad days are coming and she might start cutting.)

C: I try and not cut and I have stopped myself a few times. It's just that it keeps me from sinking further into the depression for a while.
T: Where do you cut?
C: A little below my stomach. I have an area that I cut that no one can see unless I don't have on any clothes. I wanted to do it on my arms, but I thought it was too obvious and my parents would quickly notice it.
T: I see. How big is the area you are cutting?
C: It's really very small. I don't do it often. I don't want you to think I am doing it all the time …
T: Yes, but to be able to cut in such a small place it must take some kind of skill.
C: I don't know about that. I just try to keep it hidden.
T: Sure. But to keep it hidden in such a small place that no one can see requires you to have some kind of visual or spatial skill. I don't know if I could do that in such an efficient and organized way.
C: Yeah, I just have to focus on staying within a certain area.
T: That is what I mean … you seem to have some kind of a gift at controlling how to work on something in such a small space. I think if you were cutting often you would have to figure out how to position the cuts so that they are in an order that stays hidden, but also fulfills the goal of cutting.
C: I guess …
T: How did you learn to be so precise in your work?

(Here I am capitalizing on the client's ability to do work in a small area and her skill in visual/spatial organization. Even though her cutting is not a desirable action, her intention behind it is to relieve her depression and feelings of emptiness. To initially pounce on her cutting and label it as something horrific and something to be eradicated could set up an entrenched set of actions within her initial theme. This will solidify where she is and will not help her to move out of her problem-oriented theme and its associated actions.)

C: I don't know … I don't think about it.
T: So it is a natural thing for you to do?
C: I guess, I mean I don't really have to think about it.

T: That's so fascinating to me!
C: Really?
T: Yes! Hear me out. I think that for you to be able to perform that kind of action in the way you are doing, it tells me that you have a natural ability. Maybe an ability that is not being properly used.
C: I don't understand.
T: What I mean is that it may be possible that the action of cutting at a specific place at a specific time in a specific way could be showing us that you are not allowing your natural visual and spatial intelligence to shine through.
C: But I don't want to cut ...
T: Oh, I don't want you to have to do that either. I don't want you to hurt yourself in any way, but I am wondering if this ability to be so precise in this kind of thing is a skill that many others don't have?
C: I don't know.
T: You know, I have worked with many people who cut themselves. Many of them suffer from something similar to what you have described. I have noticed that most of them do not cut themselves with the precision and detail which you demonstrate. It is like they cut for the similar reasons, but there is no thought for the spatial distance that you show. I mean, how is it that you know just the right way to stay within that special small area of the body? It is really interesting to me ... it is almost like a part of you knows just how to geometrically cut yourself to avoid serious harm to yourself and avoid being discovered. Have you ever done any kind of graphic arts work?
C: No ... well, I'm not sure. What is that?
T: I guess it could be anything ranging from stuff like painting or photography ... computer-related graphics ... maybe interior design.
C: I did used to like to paint.
T: Really?
C: Yeah, but I haven't done it in a while. I used to sketch in class. Probably more like doodle. I would draw cartoon characters a lot.
T: Wow, you see ... you have some artistic stuff going on. What classes are you taking at the college?
C: Mostly core classes. I don't really know what I want to major in yet.
T: Art?

C: No, my mother wants me to go into nursing or become a pharmacist because they are stable jobs. My father just wants me to do something practical.
T: You said your mother is a nurse. What does your father do?
C: He is an engineer. I think he is called a structural engineer.
T: OK. So he is really a practical guy.
C: Oh yes! [*Laughs*]
T: And it is natural that he wants you to do something practical.
C: Yes. He and my mother want me to be able to support myself.
T: Are you interesting in nursing?
C: I mean … it would be good to help people.
T: That doesn't sound like a glowing endorsement of your going into nursing.
C: [*Laughs*] I guess not. I mean … I would like to be open to it ….
T: I get it. What about pharmacist?
C: I guess I could do that ….
T: Another glowing endorsement?
C: It is a good and stable job, but I don't know if I would like it.
T: OK.
C: I want to do something practical …
T: You sound like Dad.
C: Yeah, but it is important to have a good career.
T: Certainly.
C: I just … I guess I just don't know …
T: Can I ask you a personal question?
C: Yes.
T: Do you ever feel that, even though you really love your parents, they just don't quite see the world the way you do? I mean, they are wonderful people who are supportive and all, but they just may have different ideas about life than you?
C: I would agree with that.
T: It is like they are both practical. They are pragmatists.
C: Yeah.
T: And you are a little different …
C: Yes.
T: You are more … Open … and artistic minded?

C: Maybe …
T: It is like you are naturally more emotional and are more in your heart and they are more in their head?
C: Yes, that true.
T: And it is great to be in your head for problem-solving and practical things, but they sometimes can't relate to you because you are in your heart? I may be wrong here, but you …
C: No, you aren't wrong. That sounds like us.
T: OK. You love them and they love you …
C: Yes.
T: … but they don't quite get you sometimes?
C: Yeah. It is like they can't understand.
T: And maybe telling them about how you have been feeling might not go well because they can't understand?
C: Yes. They would probably tell me to get over it or take medication.
T: Sure, because those are practical ways, right?
C: Yes.
T: But not everything in the world is practical, is it? Not everything is in the head. It can be in the heart sometimes too …
C: Yes.
T: It is like your parents have the head of the practical and you have the heart.
C: In a way … yes.
T: It is like you have the heart of an artist and sometimes you are surrounded by the heads of the practical.
C: It feels that way sometimes.
T: Sure. I am wondering if perhaps you have not been paying enough attention to the heart lately. It sounds like maybe you have been so focused on practical things that you haven't nurtured your artistic side. I am thinking that if you are able to do such precise visual and spatial work when you cut, maybe you also need to be doing something to nurture that talent? Some kind of artistic work … maybe that is just for you.
C: You know, when you said interior design earlier it made me think of how much I like watching all the home design and renovation shows that are on television.

114   TRANSFORMING THEMES

T: What do you like about those?
C: I like seeing the before and after of when they design or remodel a house. I really like to see how they put certain colors together and how they arranged the flow of the house.
T: You see? [*Laughs*] I told you that you had a natural artsy ability!
C: I don't know about that, but I do like seeing those changes in the homes.
T: I wonder if you need to do more artistic things to get that part of you, that artistic part of you to come through more often.
C: I don't know where to start …
T: You could start doodling again. Are you taking classes this semester?
C: Yes.
T: How about doodling a little in classes where you don't have to pay so much attention?
C: I do a little of that …
T: Do you see? It is trying to come out in you.
C: What?
T: That heart of an artist. It is trying to come out in you. I hear that you really like to watch the home decorating and improvement programs, you doodle … those kinds of things.
C: Yeah.

(The client is starting to accept the new theme of the therapy session, "The Heart of an Artist.")

T: When you don't allow yourself to explore your visual and spatial side, it is like your body takes over and does it for you in ways you don't like. It is almost as if you are trying to find something to help you open up more to the artistic realm.
C: Yeah.
T: Listen, I am going to be really, really blunt with you. You may not want to hear this and you may even want to get up and walk out that door when you hear it …
C: Uh oh. [*Laughs*] OK.
T: I think that the real problem here may be that you are really suffering from a lack of creative exploration rather than just depression. I think you may naturally feel more emotion than other people that

you know because you have been given this heart of an artist. Think about it, it is the artist that pulls from her emotions to create art. Great artists throughout history have always been a little misunderstood and had more emotions going on with them than practical people. I wonder if constantly trying to keep yourself from feeling bad and you not doing creative artistic things is making this situation worse?

C: I don't know. I just feel so overwhelmed sometimes.
T: I get it. And isn't it interesting that when you feel overwhelmed that you start doing something that requires visual and spatial precision? It is like you are trying to satisfy that visual and spatial need in you, but you are only giving yourself one option.
C: Yeah … I hadn't thought about it like that.
T: Tell me, when was the last time you really, truly gave yourself permission to tune into that heart of an artist?
C: I guess it has been a while.
T: How long?
C: I don't know … maybe … I'm just not sure.
T: If you can't be sure perhaps it has been too long. Are you willing to do something for me?
C: What?
T: I am being really serious when I ask you to do this.
C: OK.
T: I need you to go today to the local art supply place and buy something.
C: What do I buy?
T: Anything that jumps out to you as something that can kick in your artsy side. I am dead serious about this, OK?
C: OK.
T: Could you leave and do it right after our session?
C: I guess I could. I don't have to be home for a few hours.
T: Great! I wonder what kind of things might jump out at you in that store?
C: I'm not sure.
T: [*Laughs*] Me neither!
C: I haven't been to get any kind of art things in a long time.
T: Sure.

C: I won't know what to get.
T: Yeah, because right now you are trying to be practical, you know, in the head …
C: Right …
T: … and I think it will be the heart that makes the decision at the store. It will be as if a part of you will rise up to let you know, even if it doesn't make any sense.
C: I guess I could buy some new colored pencils …
T: You see? It is already letting you know. The heart is trying to get your attention. I wonder if there is something related to art that you could study at college …
C: I don't know if I could make a living being an artist.
T: Yeah, it would be tough, but I was just kind of thinking out loud if there was something practical that could also be artistic. Do you like working with computers?
C: I'm fairly good with computers. When something technical is not working at home my mother usually asks me or my father to fix it.
T: I wonder about all this graphic arts stuff and computers. I mean there are a lot of artsy jobs out there that may not sound artsy. Like advertising, marketing, architecture … you know things like that. They have to have some kind of artistic thinking as well as practical.
C: I don't know. I haven't thought about it before …
T: Because you have been in the head of the practical?
C: [*Laughs*] Maybe so.
T: I think that if you start giving yourself permission to listen to that heart of the artist you may find that the way you look at things changes. Have you ever taken any art classes in the past?
C: I took a six-week painting class during the summer when I was in middle school.
T: Did you like it?
C: Yes.
T: What kind of painting?
C: We just did oil painting of flowers. Simple things …
T: Maybe you ought to think about checking into an art class for fun?
C: I don't know. I am kind of busy now.
T: I am sure you are busy with taking care of grandma, working, school … Does grandma paint?

C: I don't think so.
T: Hmmm ... I wonder if she would like to paint.
C: I don't know.
T: If it turned out that grandma was open to painting, would you be interested in painting with her? I mean since you are already going over to her place so much.
C: Yeah ... I guess I would if she wanted to paint.
T: That might be fun.
C: Yeah.
T: OK. So you will go to the art supply store today?
C: Yes.
T: Will you do me a big favor?
C: I guess ...
T: Will you call me later and tell me what you bought?
C: Yeah.
T: Seriously.
C: Sure.
T: If I am not available leave a message with the receptionist. You can just tell her that you bought colored pencils or whatever. It will just satisfy my curiosity for what that heart of yours decides to buy.
C: OK.
T: Thank you.
C: I will.
T: Great. I think at this point you need to go ahead and see what happens at the store. Let's check back within a week or two to see what is new, if you are up for it?
C: Yeah, sure.
T: OK. Great.

Miriam left the office and called two hours later to inform me that she had purchased some colored pencils and a new sketch book. When she returned to her next therapy session two weeks later, she shared with me that she had started drawing regularly again. She also reported that, while at the art supply store, she had checked into taking painting lessons. She had mentioned this to her grandmother who told Miriam that she also wanted to take a painting class. Miriam decided that they could take a painting class together once a week. Miriam also stated that she had started looking into college programs that had an artistic aspect to them. She had even downloaded information about an art college that was a few hours away from her home. She stated that she was having fewer periods of feeling depressed, but when they did come, she found that drawing aided her in distracting herself from her symptoms. She also stated that she had not cut herself over the past two weeks.

In time, Miriam eventually decided to investigate the field of graphic arts as a career. She also found that even though she still had some periods of depression, she believed these periods were there to remind her to seek creative activities. She did not cut herself throughout the six months we worked together. Miriam told me that cutting did not do for her what her drawing did. She decided to get more involved with the local artist community and found she was really enjoying interacting with her grandmother in their art classes. She also discovered that she was talking more about personal things to her grandmother who turned out, according to Miriam, to be an "excellent therapist."

CHAPTER 7

The eccentric professor

This session is with Martin, a twenty-five-year-old man, who came to therapy presenting complaints of anxiety, depression, and a previous diagnosis of schizophrenia. When first meeting Martin, I noticed that he spoke with a very precise, but slightly robotic diction and was fairly rigid in his mannerisms.

[C = Client | T = Therapist]

T: It's nice to meet you.
C: It's nice to meet you.
T: How can I help you today?
C: Yes, I have recently moved from New York and I am looking for a therapist here.
T: When did you move here?
C: About two months ago.
T: What brought you from New York?
C: I wanted to be closer to my aunt who lives here. My mother is having some health problems and I didn't want to have to stay with her. I didn't want to be a burden.

T: So you were living with your mother?
C: Yes.
T: Why do you think you were a burden?
C: Because of my mental illness. Several years ago I was diagnosed with schizophrenia. I also had a mental breakdown four years ago which has kept me from working or going to school. I ended up having to move in with my mother. I tried to not bother my mother, but I think that my being around her so much might make her worry more about me than she needs to do.
T: I see, so you thought moving in with your aunt would help your mother?
C: Yes.
T: That is very considerate of you. Where is your father?
C: He passed away fifteen years ago from a heart attack.
T: I'm sorry to hear that.
C: My mother remarried to a nice man named Jerry. I didn't want to have to stay with them, but after my breakdown I couldn't work or live on my own. When my aunt offered for me to move in with her I thought it was an opportunity to give them some space. It was also a way for me to try and do something different.
T: You must care a lot about your mother to think about her having more space.
C: I do. She had begun to have some problems with her heart and I thought my living there with her and Jerry might be a little stressful so I moved down to be with my aunt. She has lived here for several years. She moved from New York to take a job here.
T: How has it been for you to be living down here now?
C: I don't know anyone other than my aunt. I live in a small neighborhood and occasionally see other people. They usually wave at me if they see me outside. I didn't have too many friends up in New York so I am used to being alone a lot. It gets very hot down here and it is very humid.
T: Yeah, welcome to the South!
C: [*Laughs*] Yes, it is hot. My aunt is nice to me and I appreciate her offer for me to live with her.
T: You said you had been diagnosed with schizophrenia? Is that why you have come to see me?

C: No. I have been able to manage my symptoms with my medication. I am trying to find a new psychiatrist down here to make sure that my medications are still helping. I had a psychiatrist in New York who also had me see a therapist which helped.
T: I understand. So you are saying that you are not seeking help with your schizophrenia?
C: Correct. I am coming to see you to deal with some of the anxiety and depression I feel.
T: OK.

(Martin appears to zone out and stare into space for a moment.)

T: Martin? Are you alright?
C: Yes.
T: OK.
C: I feel like I need to have both a psychiatrist and a therapist.
T: Right, I understand.
C: With my schizophrenia I sometimes have auditory and visual hallucinations.
T: Do you know when you are having those?
C: Yes, I am aware when they happen.
T: I noticed that after you told me you had come to see me because of the anxiety that you looked over into space and seemed a little agitated for a moment. Were you having a hallucination then?
C: Yes. I saw someone who I see now and then. I know it's a hallucination and I just try to ignore it.
T: Are the hallucinations frightening?
C: No. They usually last just a moment or two.
T: It must be challenging dealing with that …
C: It is, but since I started medication I have them less and they do not last as long. I have learned to know that they are not real. Many times other people don't notice when I have them. I don't say anything. I just notice them and they disappear.
T: I'm very glad to hear that they aren't frightening. I have worked with some clients who have had hallucinations that really scare them.
C: No. They aren't scary, but they can be a problem for other people who learn that I have them.

T: What usually happens when they learn that you have hallucinations?
C: Many of them stop interacting with me. My mother told me that they may get frightened, even if I don't say anything about it. I have a couple of friends who know and are fine with it, but they have usually seen me when I am doing well and not having too many of them.
T: When did you start having these hallucinations?
C: I think I was around fifteen years old. I would see things and think other people could see them. I have learned to not say too much about them around other people. My mother took me to a psychiatrist when I was seventeen and I was given some medication which helped to decrease how often they occur. I got better and then went to college for a year and a half. I then had a nervous breakdown in which I had trouble dealing with my life. I felt overwhelmed by depression and my hallucinations became worse. I had to drop out of college which I hated doing. I wanted to finish school.
T: What were you studying in school?
C: I was working on a degree in mathematics.
T: You're good in math?
C: Yes, I love math. I wanted to major in physics because of the math. I wanted to become a theoretical physicist.
T: Theoretical physics? That is pretty serious stuff.
C: I like learning about the different theories and ideas.
T: Do you think you will ever go back to college?
C: I don't know. I would very much like to go back, but I wonder if I will ever improve enough to be able to attend classes again.
T: It sounds like you miss being in college.
C: Yes. I miss the learning. I love mathematics and most science-related courses.
T: So you were unable to finish your degree?
C: No, I was not able to finish. I wanted to get a degree in mathematics and then go to graduate school for physics. I like learning about math and sometimes I feel pretty bad because I don't feel I can go back to school. Sometimes I get down because I feel like I am a burden on my family. I can't do much to help financially. I am on disability right now so I have a little bit of money to help my aunt out with the bills, but I don't feel I can work with my mental illness. I still hope that if

I find a good psychiatrist I can get the right medications to help me get a little better.
T: Have you talked to your aunt about you feeling like a burden?
C: Yes. She told me that in some ways having me live with her is a burden, but she also said she always wants to help out our family. I appreciate her letting me come and live here.

(At this point, Martin again stares off into space for a moment.)

T: Did you have another hallucination just now?
C: Yes. It usually doesn't happen so much.
T: OK. I wouldn't have known if you hadn't told me earlier that you experience those.
C: It wasn't anything bad.
T: Do you think that being unable to go to college right now and feeling like you're a burden is causing some of the anxiety and depression?
C: Yes, I do. I have had anxiety for most of my life. I also have had depression. It wasn't something that caused me problems until I had my breakdown while I was in college. The medication I started taking when I was around seventeen seemed to help some of my anxiety. I don't remember what it was. I think I feel more anxiety and depression because I am not able to do much and I feel like I am a failure because I couldn't finish school. Like I said, I don't want to burden people with my problems.

(Our first theme has emerged which we can label, "The Schizophrenic Who Is a Burden." Any disputing of Martin's perceptions of being a burden and not being able to go to college will not work in shifting the theme because this is factual information. Too much attention on the problem theme may freeze the session into an interaction that continues to perpetuate the problematic theme.)

T: I can understand that. It does sound like your aunt must on some level like having you there. Do you help out around the house?
C: Yes. I clean and help with some cooking. My aunt leaves me a daily list of things to do. I think she knows I get bored.

T: So you are giving her free maid and cook services? I bet that saves her time and money.
C: Yes. I had not thought of it like that.
T: That is why I wondered if on some level she likes you being there.
C: Yes.
T: Tell me a little more about your interest in math. I find it very interesting that you enjoy that.

(Here I am utilizing a resource that I have picked up from Martin, his love of mathematics. Anytime a client presents a potential resource, it needs to be explored in the session.)

C: Yes. I have always enjoyed math. When I was in elementary school I liked to do math drills with multiplication tables.
T: What is it about math you like so much?
C: I feel that math gives an order to the world. When you use math you have a sense of certainty about whatever it is that you are studying. I enjoy learning about physics as well. The math involved in it is interesting to me. There are many things in physics that help explain how things operate. I am also interested in the area of quantum mechanics which is different from some areas of physics.
T: I have heard of quantum mechanics. It sounds like it is very complex to me.
C: It can be, but in some ways the ideas are simple.
T: Really? What do you find simple in it?
C: Its concepts are simple, but to understand quantum mechanics can be challenging. In traditional physics, electrons exist at specific locations. In quantum mechanics, there are not specifics, but rather probabilities. It was found that certain things, such as light, can sometimes act as a particle and sometimes act as a wave. This led physicists to the conclusion that matter, which they originally saw as a particle, can also behave as a wave. Quantum mechanics is an approach used to predict the probabilities of particles. The tools used in quantum mechanics to study these things are the same as those in traditional physics. I guess what is difficult to understand is that since, at the microscopic level, matter is neither waves nor

particles, it occupies a strange area that can be localized, but also has frequency spanning over space.
T: Wow! You really enjoy this stuff don't you?

(At this point, I clearly see that Martin has an aptitude for math and physics and that he enjoys explaining the topic. By continuing to encourage discussion of his interests I am giving him a way to begin exiting out of his theme of "The Schizophrenic Who Is a Burden.")

C: Yes, it's fascinating to me.
T: I am trying to understand what you just told me. I am afraid some of those things go over my head. I really admire your ability to understand, remember, and discuss those kind of things.
C: I like breaking theories down into ways that everyone can understand.
T: You are a natural teacher.
C: I used to want to be a physics teacher when I was younger.
T: I think that you would be very good at that. The way you just summed up quantum mechanics is remarkable to me. It may be easy for people who are naturally gifted in math like yourself, but for many of us we struggle to understand those kind of complex subjects.
C: It can be complex, but the main idea is fairly simple. The quantum field is a difficult one for physicists to work in because it is difficult to predict with complete certainty the outcome of experiments. When a prediction is made in an experiment, it has to take the structure of a probability in each of the experiment's potential outcomes. This varying degree of probability led to the idea that particles can be in different states at the same time. Physicists can only predict the probability of the state that it will be in when it is measured. This can be challenging and frustrating. I think it is very interesting.
T: I can really tell that these kind of subjects fascinate you. You know what? I am really envious of you.
C: Why?
T: Because you just seem to naturally understand these kind of subjects. A lot of people would just not be able to follow them like you. You are also a natural at explaining this stuff. That is a gift.

C: I think that math is something that more people could understand if they took the time …
T: Or had a good teacher?
C: Yes.
T: I think that would be you.
C: I wanted to be a teacher …
T: Well, you are. You might not teach in a classroom, but you certainly are good at teaching me here now. I get lost on the probabilities and waves …
C: It isn't too difficult if you understand the math.
T: Which I don't. [*Laughs*]
C: If you take time it might make more sense …
T: Have you ever thought about teaching or tutoring people in math?
C: I don't have a degree in …
T: You don't need one to tutor people. I am sure there are people who need a little help somewhere and would be delighted to have someone like you take the time to explain things.
C: No, I have not done that. My mental illness can be a problem when interacting with others and …
T: So you are hesitant to approach others?
C: Yes.
T: I get it, but you know what? I am beginning to wonder if you are more like some of those eccentric and wacky professors who teach science and math in the big universities. Many of them are a little strange, yet they are able to teach and help people. They are able to take the time to coach their students. You know what I mean?
C: I think so. I had a professor who always wore a parrot tie in class.
T: A parrot tie?
C: Yes, every day he had a tie with a parrot on it.
T: Yeah! He sounds like one of those types of professors. I am wondering if you are actually a fun, eccentric professor, too. I mean eccentric in a really cool way. You see, you have these strange things that go on inside you, but yet you are a really brilliant guy who can explain complex things and make them understandable. Do you follow where I am going with this?
C: I think so.

(Now the theme is beginning to change from "The Schizophrenic Who Is a Burden" into a new theme of "The Eccentric Professor.")

T: Sure, I mean think about the really brilliant scientists that were a little weird. Look at Albert Einstein. He never combed his hair and he never wore socks. He never learned to drive. He also couldn't remember his own phone number and would get lost most days when he was trying to go home.
C: I had heard that.
T: He was a weird and eccentric guy, but he was so brilliant. I am sure you have heard of Nikola Tesla?
C: Of course.
T: He was terrified of germs and was so obsessive compulsive about everything. I had also read somewhere that at one time he believed that he might be communicating with extraterrestrials. I mean that is pretty eccentric, isn't it?
C: Yes.
T: I mean, he would have had multiple mental health diagnoses, but what a brilliant guy. Maybe you are kind of like that, a little eccentric, but able to help people understand math-related things easily?
C: I don't know.
T: Martin, I seriously think you have a gift and maybe you aren't using it as you could be. Maybe you have the ability to help people to learn math and science in a way that their traditional teachers don't. Perhaps you are that eccentric professor who helps people who are struggling with math and helps them to take their time to learn it more effectively.

(At this point, Martin is slightly nodding his head. He is looking up at the ceiling as if he is processing what has been said.)

T: Have you ever thought of offering tutoring to people in this area?
C: I haven't.
T: It might be something to think about because I wonder if you could help someone.
C: I don't have a degree in math.
T: I know, but you have this eccentric professor persona going for you.

C: [*Laughs*] Maybe I do.
T: Of course you do, but it is in a really cool way. Look, I'm not trying to tell you what to do, but I know that you have a lot to offer people. I doubt Tesla would have been able to hold down too many traditional jobs with all his problems, but he really helped transform our world.
C: He did.
T: How do you think you could use your gifts to help others? I mean, you are really good at teaching this math stuff, and I …
C: Not sure.
T: … think it could come in good use.
C: I just don't know anyone here. I have a couple of people I know in New York, but not here.
T: I get it. How about doing a recording of a math lecture?
C: I don't understand.
T: You know, make a video of you teaching something basic about math that you can share with people.
C: Who would I share it with?
T: Maybe you could send it to your mother and Jerry and those people you know in New York to start with … maybe others later.
C: Do you mean like on social media?
T: If you wanted to do that …
C: I haven't thought about doing a recording.
T: Today people are doing them with their phones. I am not saying you have to do this, but I wonder if you were to make a short video teaching something math-related. I mean, who knows?
C: Yes. I guess I could do that and just post it to people I know.
T: Sure. It might be fun to play with it. You can even watch yourself as the eccentric math professor that everyone wants to learn from …
C: My mother is usually calling to check on me. Maybe I could send her a video to show her that I am doing OK.
T: Yeah, and you can throw a little math in there … whether she likes it or not.
C: [*Laughs*] My mother is not very good in math.
T: Maybe she will watch the video and learn something?
C: Maybe.
T: How soon can you do this?
C: The video?

T: Yes.
C: I could probably do it tomorrow when my aunt is at work. I don't know what to talk about in it.
T: What area do you think basic math students tend to have issues?
C: That's easy. Fractions! I can't tell you how many people I have talked to get lost with fractions.

(At this point in the session, Martin starts to smile more and becomes noticeably more relaxed and intrigued with the idea of being an eccentric professor.)

T: That's it! You could do a fraction video as the eccentric professor. You could teach your mother and whomever else how to do basic fractions in the easy and simple way that works.
C: OK.
T: Will you do this video, Professor?
C: Yes.
T: I know it may sound a little silly, but I really feel that you need to make this video. I feel that you have a wonderful gift that is hidden away and needs to be shown. I am sure that what you do can be a benefit to those who struggle with math. I think you just need a little practice teaching and this video is good practice.
C: OK. How long should the video be?
T: I think as long as you feel it needs to be to be able to teach the basic idea you want to get across.
C: Yes. I think maybe ten minutes.
T: Great. Will you do this tomorrow and then let me know how it went when you come in for our next session?
C: Yes. I'll do it.
T: Excellent, Professor!
C: I will do it on fractions.
T: Good. I am excited to hear how the video comes out.

For the rest of the session Martin and I discussed how to record his video and how he was going to send it to other people. It was decided that he would only initially share it with people he knew who had his best interests at heart and would be a positive source of feedback. I even joked with Martin that he might need to wear some eccentric clothes to make sure everyone knew he was an eccentric professor. Before Martin left the session he had a clear plan of what to record on the video, how to send it to others, and whom to send it to for feedback. He was to return in two weeks for his next session.

Unfortunately, Martin would not return to see me further. He had to cancel his next appointment because he had been able to get an appointment with a psychiatrist at a local community mental health center earlier than he had expected and rescheduled our next session. The next week Martin called to inform me that he would be unable to continue our therapy sessions due to the community mental health center's policy which required him to see their therapists if he was using their psychiatrists. He told me he was disappointed because he felt we had worked well together, but he really needed to stay with his new psychiatrist.

Before we ended our call, Martin excitedly told me that he had made a video and sent it to his mother and stepfather along with two people he knew in New York. He said the feedback he received from them was very positive so he shared his video on his social media page. He stated that he received some positive remarks and he felt that he had helped some people understand how to do fractions better. He then told me that a couple of days later he had met a woman who lives in his neighborhood at the neighborhood mailboxes. It turned out that in talking to her he learned that her son needed some help with his math homework. Martin told me that he mustered up the courage to offer his services and let the woman know that he was a little eccentric, but he might be able to help her son with his math. The woman agreed and told Martin that she was not good at math and had a hard time explaining things to her son.

Martin told me that he had started working with the woman's son once a week and was enjoying being a math tutor. Another parent in the neighborhood had found out about Martin's tutoring and had come by his aunt's house to ask if he would be interested in also helping her child. Martin sounded very pleased with this turn of events and told me that he did not feel as anxious or depressed as he did the day he had come to see me. He also told me he was planning to make some more videos to share with others. Before our call ended, I told him that I was happy for him and that I was glad I got to meet an eccentric professor. Martin chuckled and then told me about a good book to read to help me understand quantum mechanics before he said goodbye.

References

Adler, A. (1930). Individual psychology. In: C. Murchison (Ed.), *International University Series in Psychology. Psychologies of 1930* (pp. 395–405). Worcester, MA: Clark University Press.

Bacon, S. (2018). *Practicing Psychotherapy in Constructed Reality: Ritual, Charisma, and Enhanced Client Outcomes*. Lanham, MD: Lexington.

Bateson, G. (1972). *Steps to an Ecology of the Mind*. San Francisco, CA: Chandler.

Bateson, G. (1979). *Mind and Nature: A Necessary Unity*. New York: Dutton.

Bateson, G., Jackson, D., Haley, J., & Weakland, J. (1956). Toward a theory of schizophrenia. *Behavioral Science*, *1*: 251–264.

Beck, A. T. (1993). Cognitive therapy: Nature and relation to behavior therapy. *Journal of Psychotherapy Practice and Research*, *2*: 345–356.

Bohart, A. C., & Tallman, K. (1999). *How Clients Make Therapy Work: The Process of Active Self-healing*. Washington, DC: American Psychological Association.

Carvalho, C. (2015). Therapeutic intervention and high-order adjustments of recursion. *Journal of Sociocybernetics*, *13*(2): 1–33.

Chmielewski, M., Clark, L. A., Bagby, R. M., & Watson, D. (2015). Method matters: Understanding diagnostic reliability in DSM-IV and DSM-5. *Journal of Abnormal Psychology*, *124*(3): 764–769.

Cole, V. L. (2003). Healing principles: A model for the use of ritual in psychotherapy. *Counseling and Values, 47*(3): 184–194.

Crabtree, A. (1993). *From Mesmer to Freud: Magnetic Sleep and the Roots of Psychological Healing.* New Haven, CT: Yale University Press.

Crockett, S. A., & Prosek, E. A. (2013). Promoting cognitive, emotional, and spiritual client change: The infusion of solution-focused counseling and ritual therapy. *Counseling and Values, 58*(2): 237–253.

Dowbiggin, I. R. (2009). High anxieties: the social construction of anxiety disorders. *Canadian Journal of Psychiatry, 54*(7): 429–436.

Duncan, B. L., Miller, S. D., Wampold, B. E., & Hubble, M. A. (2010). *The Heart and Soul of Change: Delivering What Works in Therapy* (2nd edn.). Washington, DC: American Psychological Association.

Ellis, A. (1994). *Reason and Emotion in Psychotherapy: A Comprehensive Method of Treating Human Disturbances: Revised and Updated.* New York: Citadel.

Farley, N. (2017). Improvisation as a meta-counseling skill. *Journal of Creativity in Mental Health, 12*(1): 115–128.

Fisch, R., Weakland, J. H., & Segal, L. (1982). *The Tactics of Change: Doing Therapy Briefly.* San Francisco, CA: Jossey-Bass.

Flemons, D. (2002). *Of One Mind: The Logic of Hypnosis, The Practice of Therapy.* New York: W. W. Norton.

Freud, S., & Breuer, J. (1895d). *Studies on Hysteria.* New York: Basic Books Classics, 2000.

Galvez, Z., & Crouch, B. (2017). Developing resilience with the improviser's mindset: Getting people out of their stuck places. In: T. Marks-Tarlow, D. J. Siegel, & M. Solomon (Eds.), *Play and Creativity in Psychotherapy (Norton Series on Interpersonal Neurobiology)* (pp. 309–337). New York: W. W. Norton.

Gergen, K. (2009). *An Invitation to Social Construction.* London: Sage.

Goodwyn, E. D. (2016). *Healing Symbols in Psychotherapy: A Ritual Approach.* New York: Routledge.

Gordon, D., & Meyers-Anderson, M. (1981). *Phoenix: Therapeutic Patterns of Milton H. Erickson.* Capitola, CA: Meta.

Greenberg, R. P. (2016). The rebirth of psychosocial importance in a drug filled world. *American Psychologist, 71*(8): 781–791.

Hale, D., & Frusha, C. V. (2016). MRI brief therapy: A tried and true systemic approach. *Journal of Systemic Therapies, 35*(2): 14–24.

Haley, J. (1987). *Problem Solving Therapy.* San Francisco, CA: Jossey-Bass.

Haley, J. (1993). *Jay Haley on Milton H. Erickson*. Bristol, PA: Brunner/Mazel.

Hogue, D. A. (2006). Healing of the self-in-context: Memory, plasticity, and spiritual practice. In: J. Koss-Chioino & P. J. Hefner (Eds.), *Spiritual Transformation and Healing: Anthropological, Theological, Neuroscientific, and Clinical Perspectives* (pp. 223–238). Lanham, MD: AltaMira.

Horwitz, A. V. (2011). Creating an age of depression: The social construction and consequences of the major depression diagnosis. *Society and Mental Health*, *1*(1): 41–54.

Johansen, R., Iversen, V. C., Melle, I., & Hestad, K. A. (2013). Therapeutic alliance in early schizophrenia spectrum disorders: A cross-sectional study. *Annals of General Psychiatry*, *12*(1): 14.

Jung, C. G. (1960). *On the Nature of the Psyche*. New York: Bollingen Foundation.

Keeney, B. P. (1983). *Aesthetics of Change*. New York: Guilford.

Keeney, H., Keeney, B., & Chenail, R. (2015). *Recursive Frame Analysis: A Qualitative Research Method for Mapping Change-oriented Discourse*. Ft. Lauderdale, FL: The Qualitative Report Books.

Kirmayer, L. J. (1993). Healing and the invention of metaphor: the effectiveness of symbols revisited. *Culture, Medicine and Psychiatry*, *17*(2): 161–195.

Korzybski, A. (1958). *Science and Sanity: An Introduction to Non-Aristotelian Systems and General Semantics*. Brooklyn, NY: Institute of General Semantics.

Krippendorff, K. (1984). An epistemological foundation of communication. *Journal of Communication*, *34* (3): 21–36.

Leslie, P. J. (2014). *Potential Not Pathology: Helping Your Clients Transform Using Ericksonian Psychotherapy*. New York: Routledge.

Neuman, Y. (2003). *Processes and Boundaries of the Mind: Extending the Limit Line*. Boston, MA: Springer.

Neuringer, C. (1992). Freud and the theatre. *Journal of the American Academy of Psychoanalysis*, *20*(1): 142–148.

O'Hanlon, B., & Wilk, J. (1987). *Shifting Contexts: The Generation of Effective Psychotherapy*. New York: Guilford.

O'Hanlon, W. H. (1987). *Taproots: Underlying Principles of Milton Erickson's Therapy and Hypnosis*. New York: W. W. Norton.

Papp, P., & Imber-Black, E. (1996). Family themes: Transmission and transformation. *Family Process*, *35*(1): 5–20.

Poland, J. (2015). DSM-5 and research concerning mental illness. In: *The DSM-5 in Perspective* (pp. 25–42). Dordrecht, the Netherlands: Springer.

Priebe, S., Richardson, M., Cooney, M., Adedeji, O., & McCabe, R. (2011). Does the therapeutic relationship predict outcomes of psychiatric treatment in patients with psychosis? A systematic review. *Psychotherapy and Psychosomatics*, 80(2): 70–77.

Rabaté, J. M. (2002). Loving Freud madly: Surrealism between hysterical and paranoid modernism. *Journal of Modern Literature*, 25(3): 58–74.

Ray, W., & Keeney, B. (1993). *Resource Focused Therapy*. London: Karnac.

Rogers, C. R. (1946). Significant aspects of client-centered therapy. *American Psychologist*, 1: 415–422.

Rohrbaugh, M. J., & Shoham, V. (2001). Brief therapy based on interrupting ironic processes: The Palo Alto model. *Clinical Psychology: Science and Practice*, 8(1): 66–81.

Shinebourne, P. (2006). Trauma and culture: on Freud's writing about trauma and its resonances in contemporary cultural discourse. *British Journal of Psychotherapy*, 22(3): 335–345.

Short, D., Erickson, B. A., & Erickson-Klein, R. (2005). *Hope and Resiliency: Understanding the Psychotherapeutic Strategies of Milton H. Erickson. M.D.* Carmarthen, UK: Crown House.

Spencer-Brown, G. (1969). *Laws of Form*. London: Allen & Unwin.

Spolin, V. (1999). *Improvisation for the Theater: A Handbook of Teaching and Directing Techniques* (3rd edn.). Evanston, IL: Northwestern University Press.

Strupp, H. H., & Hadley, S. W. (1979). Specific vs nonspecific factors in psychotherapy: A controlled study of outcome. *Archives of General Psychiatry*, 36(10): 1125–1136.

Thomason, T. (2005). A brief history of psychotherapy. Retrieved from http://works.bepress.com/timothy_thomason/25/ (last accessed April 5, 2020).

Van Der Hart, O. (1983). *Rituals in Psychotherapy: Transition and Continuity*. New York: Irvington.

Von Foerster, H. (2003). Cybernetics of cybernetics. In: *Understanding Understanding* (pp. 283–286). New York: Springer.

Wampold, B. E. (2015). How important are the common factors in psychotherapy? An update. *World Psychiatry*, 14(3): 270–277.

Wampold, B. E., & Imel, Z. E. (2015). *The Great Psychotherapy Debate: The Evidence for What Makes Psychotherapy Work*. New York: Routledge.

Watson, J. B. (2017). *Behaviorism*. New York: Routledge.

Index

abstracting process, 6, 9
Adedeji, O., 33
Adler, A., 27
    inferiority complex, 28
adolescent and parent interaction, 7
anxiety and depression, 119
    client's anxiety, 29
    creating new theme, 125
    depression, 105–118
    "Eccentric Professor, The", 127–130
    hallucinations, 121
    issues with coping, 91–104
    resource utilization, 124
    "Schizophrenic Who Is a Burden, The", 123–127
archetypes, 28

Bacon, S., 22, 34–35, 42
Bagby, R. M., 38
Bateson, G., 4, 7, 32
Bateson Project, 31–32
Beck, A. T., 31

behavior
    ability to perceive, 4
    controlling, 27
    therapy, 29
behaviorism, 29
behavior therapy, 29
Bohart, A. C., 44
Bohart and Tallman hypothesis, 44
borderline personality, 39–42
Breuer, J., 26

Carvalho, C., 9
catalysts for seeking therapist help, 2
changing themes in therapy, 18
    see also theme-oriented therapy
Charcot, 26
Chenail, R., 8, 11
Chmielewski, M., 38
Clark, L. A., 38
clients' themes, working with, 2
cocreating new themes, 49
    being open to anything, 58–64

cocreative process, 58
emphasizing resources, 50–56
improvisation, 56–64
new theme, 50
problem-oriented themes, 49, 51
random information, 57
resistance, 67
resourceful theme, 50–51
social anxiety, 52–56
spontaneously created themes, 56
in theme-creation view, 49
utilization, 64–70
cocreative process, 58 *see also* cocreating new themes
cognition, 3–4
cognitive bias, 21
cognitive therapies, 30–31
Cole, V. L., 86
collective unconscious, 28
common factors, 33
conscious mind-oriented therapy, 72
   see also thematic pattern alterations
constructed contexts, 7
constructions, metaphoric, 87
context, 7 *see also* theme-oriented therapy
conversations, improvised, 13
conversion disorder, 26
Cooney, M., 33
couple therapy, 23
Crabtree, A., 25
Crockett, S. A., 85, 86
Crouch, B., 58
curiosity, despair to, 16

depression, 105 *see also* anxiety and depression
   capitalizing on client's ability, 110
   good and bad days, 109
   "Heart of an Artist, The", 114–118
   seeking creative activities, 117–118
   "Woman Who Wore an Iron Jacket, The", 109
diagnosing as theme creation, 36–42
diagnosis, 36
   of borderline personality, 39–42

diagnostic categories, 39
language in, 38
mental illness categories, 42
in psychotherapy, 38
Diagnostic and Statistical Manual of Mental Disorders (DSM), 38, 42
distinction(s), 2–5, 10, 19–21, 37, 56
   see also theme-oriented therapy
"dodo bird" effect, 33
Dowbiggin, I. R., 39
DSM *see Diagnostic and Statistical Manual of Mental Disorders*
Duncan, B. L., 33

effective and transformative therapy, 36
Ellis, A., 30
emotion, ability to perceive, 4
empowering themes, 12–13
Erickson, B. A., 45
Erickson, M.
   approach and method, 44–47
   use of utilization, 65
Erickson-Klein, R., 45
experiences, higher and lower-order, 10
explanatory devices, xii

family systems therapy, 31–32
   see also Haley, J.
Farley, N., 58
Fisch, R., 72
Flemons, D., 4–5
Freud, S., 26
   controversial views, 27
   vs. Jung, 28
   therapy of psychoanalysis, 26–27
Frusha, C. V., 72

Galvez, Z., 58
Gergen, K., 21–24, 37
Goodwyn, E. D., 86–87
Gordon, D., 47
Greenberg, R. P., 33
grief, show of, 13–14

Hadley, S. W., 34
Hale, D., 72

Haley, J., 32, 38, 45
hallucinations, 121
healing themes, 12–13
Hestad, K. A., 33
higher-order complexity, xiii
Hogue, D. A., 87
Horwitz, A. V., 38
Hubble, M. A., 33
humanistic psychology, 29
    therapies, 29–30
humanistic therapists, 29–30
hypnotic interventions for psychopathology, 26
hysteria, 26

Imber-Black, E., xii, 8, 10–12, 50, 56, 73, 85
Imel, Z. E., 33–34
improvisation, 56–64 *see also* cocreating new themes
improvised conversations, 13
individualized resource-directed themes, 44–47
inferiority complex, 28
interaction, parent and adolescent, 7
issues with coping, 91
    "Soldier That Was Secretly a Hippie, The", 100–104
    theme of being "bad", 95
Iversen, V. C., 33

Jackson, D., 32
Janet, P., 26
Johansen, R., 33
Jung, C. G., 28
    archetypes, 28
    mystical-tinged therapy, 28–29

Keeney, B., xiii, 8, 11–12
Keeney, B. P., 3, 5
Keeney, H., 8, 11
Kirmayer, L. J., 71, 87
Korzybski, A., 5, 21
Krippendorff, K., 3

language, 4, 22–23, 72
Leslie, P. J., 45

mammalian retina, 3
Marquis de Puységur, 25
McCabe, R., 33
meanings, 10, 19, 22, 24
    higher-order, 3, 6, 9
    ritual, 86
Melle, I., 33
mental health, medicalization, 38
mental illness, 24–25
    categories of, 42
Mesmer, F. A., 25–26
Mesmerism, 25
metaphoric constructions, 87
Meyers-Anderson, M., 47
Miller, S. D., 33
mystical-tinged therapy, 28–29

Neuman, Y., 3
Neuringer, C., 27

objective reality, 10
objectivity, 21
O'Hanlon, B., 12
O'Hanlon, W. H., 45
outer and inner personality, 91–104

Papp, P., xii, 8, 10–12, 50, 56, 73, 85
parent and adolescent interaction, 7
"Parents Who Saw Too Much, The", 15
Poland, J., 39, 42
post-traumatic stress disorder (PTSD), 40–41
predetermined therapy themes, 20
Priebe, S., 33
problem-oriented themes, 19–20, 49, 51, 85
Prosek, E. A., 85–86
psychoanalysis, theme of, 27
psychotherapy, 21, 24, 35 *see also* problem-oriented themes
    Bohart and Tallman hypothesis, 44
    role of diagnosis in, 38
    traditional therapy, 47–48
psychotherapy as theme creation, 19
    couple therapy, 23
    creating new themes, 43
    diagnosing as theme creation, 36–42

dichotomous perception of "problem/no problem", 20
fundamental reality vs. constructed reality, 22
history of psychotherapy themes, 24–36
individualized resource-directed themes, 44–47
language, 22–23
medicalization of mental health, 38
objectivity, 21
predetermined therapy themes, 20
problem-oriented theme, 19–20
psychotherapy, 21, 24
reality, maps of, 21
reproducing meaning in shared reality, 19
therapeutic theories, 21
therapy themes awareness, 43–48
verbal constructions, 22
psychotherapy themes, 24
  Bateson Project, 31–32
  behaviorism, 29
  behavior therapy, 29
  client's anxiety, 29
  cognitive therapies, 31
  common factors, 33
  controlling behavior, 27
  "dodo bird" effect, 33
  effective and transformative therapy, 36
  efficacy of professional and nonprofessional therapists, 34
  family systems therapy, 31
  Freud's therapy of psychoanalysis, 26–27
  humanistic psychology and therapies, 29–30
  hypnotic interventions for psychopathology, 26
  inferiority complex, 28
  mental illness, 24–25
  Mesmerism, 25–26
  mystical-tinged therapy, 28–29
  theme of psychoanalysis, 27
  therapeutic alliance, 33

"Toward a Theory of Schizophrenia", 32
PTSD *see* post-traumatic stress disorder

Rabate, J. M., 27
Ray, W., xiii, 12
reality
  maps of, 21
  objective, 10
  perceptions of, 5
recursion, 9
"Reluctant Preacher, The", 17
reproducing meaning in shared reality, 19
resource, 50–56 *see also* cocreating new themes
  -directed themes, 44–47
resourceful theme, 50–51
Richardson, M., 33
rituals *see* therapeutic rituals
Rogers, C. R., 30
Rohrbaugh, M. J., 72

schemas, 6
seeking therapist help, 2
Segal, L., 72
separation, mindful acts of, 4–5
Shinebourne, P., 27
shock and horror, 1
Shoham, V., 72
Short, D., 45
show of grief, 13–14
social anxiety, 52–56
Spencer-Brown, G., 3
Spolin, V., 57
spontaneously created themes, 56 *see also* cocreating new themes
staying within theme, 11
Strupp, H. H., 34
symbolic ritual, 87–88 *see also* therapeutic rituals

Tallman, K., 44
thematic pattern alterations, 71–72, 85
  see also therapeutic rituals
  adding to patterns, 82–85
  adjusting when patterns occur, 75–77
  altering duration of patterns, 80–82

altering where patterns occur, 77–80
methods of, 75
unconscious processes, 72–73
theme, xi *see also* cocreating new themes; psychotherapy as theme creation; psychotherapy themes; theme-oriented therapy
   ability to adjust, 8
   of being "bad", 95
   change in therapy, 18
   changing higher-order, 9–10
   creating new, 125
   diagnosing as creation of, 36–42
   empowering, 12–13
   individualized resource-directed, 44–47
   -oriented approach components of, 71
   -oriented theme, 19–20, 49, 51, 85
   predetermined therapy, 20
   problem-oriented, 19–20, 49, 51, 85
   resourceful, 50–51
   spontaneously created, 56
   staying within, 11
theme-oriented therapy, 1
   ability to adjust themes, 8
   ability to perceive emotion or behavior, 4
   analogy of three-act play, 12
   catalysts for seeking therapist help, 2
   changing higher-order of context/themes, 9–10
   changing themes in therapy, 18
   cognition, 3–4
   constructed contexts, 7
   context, 7
   despair to curiosity, 16
   drawing distinction, 2–4
   empowering or healing themes, 12–13
   higher-order meanings, 6
   higher order vs. lower-order experiences, 10
   improvised conversations, 13
   inferences, 10
   language, 4
   mindful acts of separation, 4–5
   objective reality, 10
   parent and male adolescent interaction, 7
   "Parents Who Saw Too Much, The", 15
   perceptions of reality, 5
   problems to larger themes, 8
   recursion, 9
   "Reluctant Preacher, The", 17
   schemas, 6
   shock and horror, 1
   show of grief, 13–14
   staying within theme, 11
   verbal level of abstracting process, 6
   word, 5
   working with clients' themes, 2
   worldviews, 2
therapeutic alliance, 33
therapeutic rituals, 71, 85–90 *see also* thematic pattern alterations
   changes by, 86
   construction of, 87
   metaphoric constructions, 87
   problem-oriented themes, 85
   purpose of, 85
   symbolic ritual, 87–88
therapeutic theories, 21
therapist efficacy, 34–36
therapy
   behavior, 29
   cognitive, 31
   couple, 23
   family systems, 31
   of Freud's psychoanalysis, 26–27
   humanistic psychology and, 29–30
   hypnotic interventions for psychopathology, 26
   themes awareness, 43–48
   transformative, 36
Thomason, T., 25
three-act play analogy, 12
"Toward a Theory of Schizophrenia", 32
traditional "talk" therapy, 71 *see also* thematic pattern alterations
transformative therapy, 36

unconscious processes, 72–73
utilization, 64–70 *see also* cocreating new themes
Van Der Hart, O., 85
verbal constructions, 22
Von Foerster, H., 21

Wampold, B. E., 33–34
Watson, D., 38
Watson, J. B., 29
Weakland, J., 32
Weakland, J. H., 72
Wilk, J., 12
word, 5
working with clients' themes, 2
worldviews, 2